Dedication/Acknowledgments

This book is dedicated to all the patients who call their doctors day after day for their never-ending pain.

I would like to thank a few people who encouraged me to write this book. First of all, I have to acknowledge my thanks to the scared, frustrated and helpless NAET patients, who call me many times during my office hours, and even at night, for some relief from their emergency health problems during their initial visits in my office.

My special thanks also go to my son Roy, and my husband Kris, who sat and worked till early hours in the mornings to formulate this book. I would also like to thank the artists and printers who did a great job on creating this book.

First edition, October 1997

Copyright© 1997

by
Devi S. Nambudripad,
D.C., L.Ac, R.N., Ph.D.
Buena Park, CA 90621

All Rights Reserved

Library of Congress Catalog Number: 97-092300
ISBN Number: 0-9658242-0-9
Printed in U.S.A.

CONTENTS

PREFACE 6

INTRODUCTION..7

HOW TO USE THE BOOK - INSTRUCTIONS 10

PART I

Chapter 1
General Description of the Traditional Chinese Acupuncture/ acupressure point Locations and Their Overall Functions.
Acupressure Techniques 11

Chapter 2
Location and common usages of the acupressure points 15

Chapter 3
Acupressure guidelines...32

Chapter 4
General balancing points...58

Chapter 5
Acupressure points without Illustrations. 59

PART II

Chapter 6
Point Illustrations 63
1.   ABDOMINAL BLOATING...64
2.   ABDOMINAL PAIN 65
3.   ABDOMINAL PAINS DUE TO OVEREATING...66
4.   ABDOMINAL SPASMS (Colic)..67
5.   LOWER ABDOMINAL PAIN...68
6.   ACUTE VIRAL INFECTION 69
7.   ACUTE APPENDICITIS 70
8.   ADHD (Attention Deficit and Hyperactive Disorder)...............................71
9.   ACNE...72
10.   ADDICTION TO FOOD, DRUGS, CAFFEINE, CHOCOLATE AND ALCOHOL.....73
11.   ANGER 74
12.   ANGIONEUROTIC EDEMA 75
13.   ANOREXIA NERVOSA..76
14.   ANXIETY ATTACKS 77
15.   ARTHRITIS OF THE FINGERS 78
16.   ARTHRITIS OF THE HAND 79

17. ARTHRITIS OF THE ELBOW 80
18. ARTHRITIS OF THE SHOULDER 81
19. ARTHRITIS OF THE WRIST 82
20. ARTHRITIS OF THE HIP JOINT 83
21. ARTHRITIS OF THE KNEE 84
22. ARTHRITIS OF THE ANKLES AND TOES 85
23. OSTEO-ARTHRITIS 86
24. RHEUMATOID ARTHRITIS 87
25. LUPUS-ARTHRITIS 88
26. ASCITES 89
27. ASTHMA 90
28. LOWER BACKACHE 91
29. MID BACKACHE 92
30. UPPER BACKACHE 93
31. BACTERIAL INFECTION 94
32. BLEEDING FROM THE GUMS 95
33. BLEEDING FROM THE NOSE 96
34. BLEEDING FROM THE EYES 97
35. BLEEDING FROM THE MOUTH 98
36. BLEEDING FROM THE MUCOUS MEMBRANES 99
37. BLEEDING FROM THE STOMACH 100
38. BLOOD DISORDERS 101
39. BLOOD IN THE STOOL 102
40. BLOOD IN THE URINE 103
41. EXCESSIVE UTERINE BLEEDING 104
42. BLEEDING FROM THE RECTUM 105
43. HEMORRHOIDS, BLEEDING OR IRRITATION 106
44. BURNING FEET 107
45. BLOCKAGE OF THE SINUSES 108
46. BLURRED VISION 109
47. BRAIN FOG 110
48. PAIN IN THE BREAST 111
49. BRONCHITIS 112
50. BULIMIA 113
51. BUTTERFLY SENSATION OR NERVOUS STOMACH 114
52. CARDIAC AND RESPIRATORY ARREST 115
53. CHEST PAINS OR CARDIAC PAINS 116
54. CELIAC SPRUE 117
55. CHEMICAL SENSITIVITY 118

56.	LUNG CONGESTION	119
57.	EMOTIONAL CHEST PAIN	120
58.	CONSTIPATION	121
59.	COLD LIMBS	122
60.	CHOKING WHILE YOU TALK TO STRANGERS (SHYNESS)	123
61.	CHRONIC FATIGUE SYNDROME	124
62.	COMA OR SEMI-CONSCIOUSNESS	125
63.	COLITIS	126
64.	COLD SORES	127
65.	COMMON COLD	128
66.	CONVULSIONS	129
67.	COUGH	130
68.	CRAMPS IN THE LEGS	131
69.	CRAMPS IN THE LOWER ABDOMEN	132
70.	CROHN'S DISEASE/IRRITABLE BOWELS	133
71.	CRYING SPELLS	134
72.	DEAFNESS AND RINGING IN THE EAR	135
73.	DEPRESSION	136
74.	DIARRHEA	137
75.	DIFFICULTY IN BREATHING	138
76.	DIFFICULTY IN SWALLOWING	139
77.	DIFFICULTY IN URINATING	140
78.	DISCOLORATION OF THE SCLERA	141
79.	DIVERTICULITIS	142
80.	DIZZINESS	143
81.	NIGHTMARES	144
82.	DRYNESS OF THE MOUTH	145
83.	DRYNESS OF THE TONGUE	146
84.	DYSENTERY	147
85.	DYSMENORRHEA	148
86.	EARACHE	149
87.	EAR INFECTION	150
88.	EATING DISORDERS	151
89.	ECZEMA	152
90.	EDEMA	153
91.	ELECTRIC AND ELECTRO-MAGNETIC ENERGY IMBALANCES	154
92.	ENVIRONMENTAL TOXICITY	155
93.	EYE INFLAMMATION	156
94.	EYE INFECTIONS	157
95.	EYE PAIN	158

96.	EYE STRESS	159
97.	EPILEPSY	160
98.	EPSTEIN-BARR VIRUS	161
99.	EXCESSIVE PERSPIRATION	162
100.	FAINTING	163
101.	FEVER	164
102.	FIBROMYALGIA	165
103.	FOOD POISONING	166
104.	GENERAL BODY ACHE	167
105.	GALL BLADDER PAIN	168
106.	HEAT STROKE	169
107.	HEAT SENSATION IN THE SOLE	170
108.	HEART IRREGULARITIES	171
109.	HYPOGLYCEMIA	172
110.	HEADACHES IN GENERAL	173
111.	MIGRAINES (GALL BLADDER HEADACHES)	174
112.	MIGRAINES (LIVER HEADACHES)	175
113.	MIGRAINES (STOMACH HEADACHES)	176
114.	MIGRAINES (BLADDER HEADACHES)	177
115.	HEARTBURN	178
116.	HIGH BLOOD PRESSURE	179
117.	HIVES	180
118.	INDIGESTION	181
119.	INSOMNIA	182
120.	LARYNGITIS	183
121.	LEAKY GUT SYNDROM	184
122.	LOW ENERGY	185
123.	MENSTRUATION TROUBLE (PMS)	186
124.	NAUSEA/Side effects of radiation and chemotherapy	187
125.	OVERACTIVE MIND	188
126.	RESTLESS LEG SYNDROME	189
127.	SCIATIC NEURALGIA	190
128.	SHORTNESS OF BREATH	191
129.	SORE THROAT	192
130.	TOOTHACHE	193
131.	UNABLE TO CRY	194
132	NERVOUSNESS OF ALL KINDS	195
BIBLIOGRAPHY		**196**
ANATOMICAL POSITIONS		**196**
INDEX		**197**
CERTIFIED NAET PRACTITIONERS		**202**
BOOKS ORDER FORM		

This book is written in two parts. Part one in five chapters, introduces the concept of acupressure and its uses in pain management. This section also helps you to locate the therapeutic pressure points in your body. Chapter three explains the benefits of these points. I believe most of our health problems arise from some form of allergy. Specific allergens cause specific health problems. We have taken most of the health problems seen in my practice and tried to organize them, so that readers, who are NAET practitioners, could benefit from this section using it for case management. By studying this book, you will not only learn how to treat with acupressure, but also learn to investigate the root of your health problems. Any condition that is not congenital or accidental in nature could be the result of an allergy. Allergens like food, drinks, clothes, cosmetics, environmental substances, pollutants, chemicals, all are equally hazardous for an allergic person. If the reader is interested about allergies, please read the book "Say Goodbye To Illness" by the author. In conclusion, I hope you will be able to utilize the knowledge in this book to your benefit and to the benefit of the others that you care about.

LIVING PAIN FREE
By Using Acupressure

Dr. Devi S. Nambudripad, D.C., L.Ac., R.N., Ph.D.

Acupressure/Acupuncture is an important part of Traditional Chinese Medicine. The origins of Traditional Chinese Medicine are not really known. It is believed to have been developed between 2500 and 4500 BC. Also, historians believe that TCM (Traditional Chinese Medicine) could have started by accumulating the knowledge about simple folk medicines from all over the country by various Chinese medical practitioners and scholars and put together by someone else who had the common interest. In those days, the people of China consisted mainly of peasants, who worked hard in the fields. When they worked in the fields for long hours they developed aches and pains. The medical practitioners experimented by massaging and pushing at certain painful points to alleviate the daily pains and discomforts of their Chinese peasant- patients. The deeply caring doctors and considerate Emperors of those times encouraged the developments and investigations of these medical practices and knowledge hoping that they would get better results with their treatments. The Emperors who ruled China took keen interest in encouraging the development of Chinese Medicine to provide a better life for their subjects. The legendary Emperors who worked to improve Traditional Chinese Medicine are "Shen Nung", "Huang Di", and "Fu shu". It is believed that these are the originators of Traditional Chinese Medicine. The classical book on Traditional Chinese Medicine is the "Huang Di Nei Jing", meaning, "The yellow Emperor's Classic of Internal Medicine," and this work is credited to "Huang Di" (The yellow Emperor), who is believed to have lived about 2697 - 2596 BC Some critics argue that TCM was not discovered entirely during this time. Some say that over a period of time, the knowledge was accumulating in the peoples' minds, waiting for someone to begin the documentation of their findings. More likely, Huang Di initiated the process of collection and compilation of data from all the pioneers until his time and gave TCM a name and a shape. From then on, people began to keep actual documentation. TCM has travelled a long way through step by step growth to reach today's standard. "Huang Di Nei Jing" is the earliest documented material historians have found so far. No other written proof of work has been discovered before this period. This book "Nei Jing" is presented as a dialogue between the Yellow Emperor and his efficient, well-versed prime minister who was also a palace physician.

This book is written in two sections.

1. **Su Wen**: contains the principles of traditional Chinese medicine and simple questions about preventive Medicine.

2. **Ling Shu**: describes the treatments and modalities for a variety of health conditions and how to take care of them.

One of the fundamental concepts of Chinese Medicine is that *Chi* is an invisible force which gives life to all living matter. If there is an obstruction to this energy flow, then the blocked area will suffer from illness. Various techniques can be used to reinstate the flow of *Chi* through the channels and collaterals of the body. Acupuncture, acupressure, manipulation, herbs, smelling salts, purging (herbal laxatives, suppositories, colonics, enemas), exercises, massages with oils (herbal oil, aromatic oils, medicinal powders, cooked grains, herbal extracts), having an insect bite the area of illness, (e.g. making a leech to suck the blood from the area), were some of the techniques used in those days to remove energy blockages and to reinstate the energy flow.

Acupressure was one of the common modalities used to achieve therapeutic effect. Acupressure can play a great role in relieving energy blockages and restart the flow of energy into the tissues and organs. When the energy flow increases, blood circulation to the area increases and when that happens, the impurities and excess fluids will move out of the area and nutrition will move in. This in turn can reduce aches and

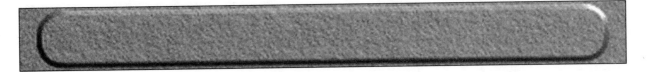

pains in a person in a short period of time. Pain and/or discomfort is the body's alarm signal. When dealing with pain, it is essential that the causes are understood. Pain may be caused by any number of factors. But when we suffer from many allergies, these allergies can cause an accumulation of toxins, unwanted chemicals in the tissues and cause pain and discomfort of various types without any further provocation. Very often, acupressure can turn off pain or render great relief from pain or discomfort in a few minutes.

Through a series of monthly patient education seminars, my patients were taught acupressure to handle most of their health emergencies. Some of these patients were in emergency rooms practically every night before they were taught acupressure self help. Now they rarely have to go to the emergency rooms or wake up their doctors in the middle of the night. I had requests from many of these patients to create a reference manual with all the points I have been teaching them through the seminars, to use as a quick reference for their future emergency needs. My patients and I strongly believe that the knowledge about these simple acupressure points can save you time, money and mental peace in your health emergencies. It is very necessary to do it right. So, please learn the correct way to get optimum results. Not doing the correct procedure is not going to cause any damage to the person. But, You may not receive the expected result. This acupressure therapy is for temporary relief only. This does not replace the need for medical practitioners. If you do not get relief by massaging these points, please contact your doctor for further help. This is a safe technique to practice on infants, children, adults, older, sick or healthy people. Very gentle massage or gentle taps with the pads (tips) of your fingers on the surface of the skin is all that is needed. Do not apply too much pressure. The therapy may not work well when you apply too much pressure. You may need to apply different methods of acupressure according to your condition and need. Please find the method that suits your need.

Devi S. Nambudripad, D.C., L.Ac, R.N., Ph.D.
Buena Park, CA 90621
(714) 523-0800
October, 1997

How to use the Book - Instructions

STEP BY STEP INSTRUCTIONS TO USE THIS BOOK

First read page 11, to learn the correct acupressure technique.

GO TO PAGES 33 - 59 to find your specific health problem. Acupoint illustrations for these conditions are given in pages 64 - 195.

More health conditions are given in pages 59 - 62 . You shall see a list of specific acupressure points written next to the condition without any acupoint illustrations.

Note down the respective acupressure points related to your disorder.

Find the acupressure charts related to the disorder in pages 64-195.

If there is no chart given for the health condition, please go to pages 13 and 14 to find the correct location of the acupressure points of your need.

Then, go to page 58 and follow the instructions to balance the body. A battery operated or electrical acupoint stimulator may be used in place of finger massage.

After balancing the body, use acupressure on the specific acupressure points to get relief from your health problem. If you are in doubt about the procedure, or seriously ill, or if your problem persists, please see a physician.

If you suffer from many allergies, please see an NAET practitioner nearest you. Some of the NAET practitioners' names and telephone numbers are given at the end of this book.

Please call 714-523-0800 for the most recent list of NAET practitioners.

CHAPTER 1

ACUPRESSURE TECHNIQUES

Acupressure points are located bilaterally (both sides of the body), except on conception vessel (CV), and governing vessel (GV) meridians.

1. **To get more energy:** This type is for the people without energy, exhaustion due to overwork, a very weak person who is recovering from a major illness (surgeries, etc.), currently suffering from an illness, poor energy due to malnutrition, poor digestion, allergies, chemical toxicity, etc.

2. **Suffering from too much energy:** Excess energy may be due to malfunctioning of adrenal glands or any other internal organ disfunction, other health conditions like hyperactivity, irritability, manic depression, food allergies, attention deficit and hyperactive disorders, etc.

3. **Pain of different types and levels:** Mild, moderate and severe amount of pain from various conditions.

4. **To improve general health:** Person without health problems wanting to improve overall general health.

Methods of Applying Acupressure

1. **To get more energy:** Gently tap using your pads of the fingers, use a point stimulator, or massage on the points for your particular problem for one half of a minute (30 seconds) on each point clockwise once or twice a day or gentle tap for 30 seconds. [Point stimulator for 15 seconds on each point].

2. **Too much energy:** Gently massage using the pads of your fingers on the appropriate set of points for your particular problem for 1-3 minutes on each point,

counter clockwise, two to four times a day. Movement of the fingers for massage from left to right in a circular fashion on the point or gentle tap on the point for 1-3 minutes. [Point stimulator for 30 seconds on each point].

3. **In case of severe pain:** Massage the appropriate points counter-clockwise for 1 minute on each point (from left to right). Repeat the cycle every five to ten minutes for six to ten times or until you get relief. In case of dull pain, massage clockwise for 1 minute on each point (from right to left, and left to right). Repeat the cycle every five to ten minutes for six to ten times or until you get relief. [Point stimulator for 30 seconds on each point].

4. **To improve general health:** Gently tap on the points or apply gentle massage clockwise for 30 seconds to 1 minute twice a day. [Point stimulator for 15 seconds on each point].

5. When you use acupressure, you may use one, two or all the points. In some cases, people may just need one pressure point to get relief.

Abbreviations:

GV =   Governing Vessel Meridian
CV =   Conception Vessel Meridian
Lu =   Lung Meridian
LI =   Large Intestine Meridian
St =   Stomach Meridian
Sp =   Spleen Meridian
Pc =   Pericardium Meridian
TH =   Triple Heater Meridian
Ht =   Heart Meridian
Liv =   Liver Meridian
GB =   Gall Bladder Meridian
Kid =   Kidney Meridian
SI =   Small Intestine Meridian
UB =   Urinary Bladder Meridian

Finger measurement: When the middle finger is flexed, the distance between the two ends of the creases of the interphalangeal joints is taken as one body inch. Four finger breadths = three body inches.

If you want more detail information about Acupuncture/Acupressure meridians, please read the reference books (3), (5) in the bibliography.

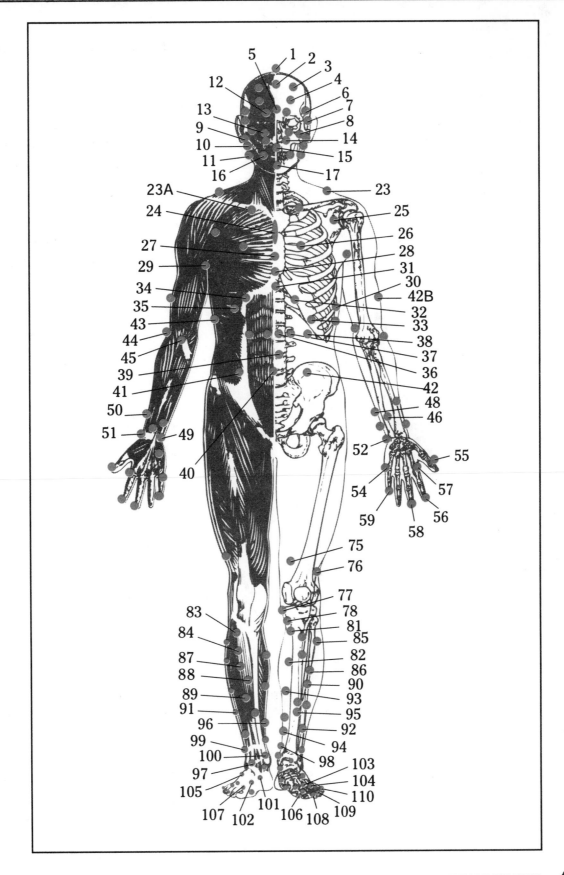

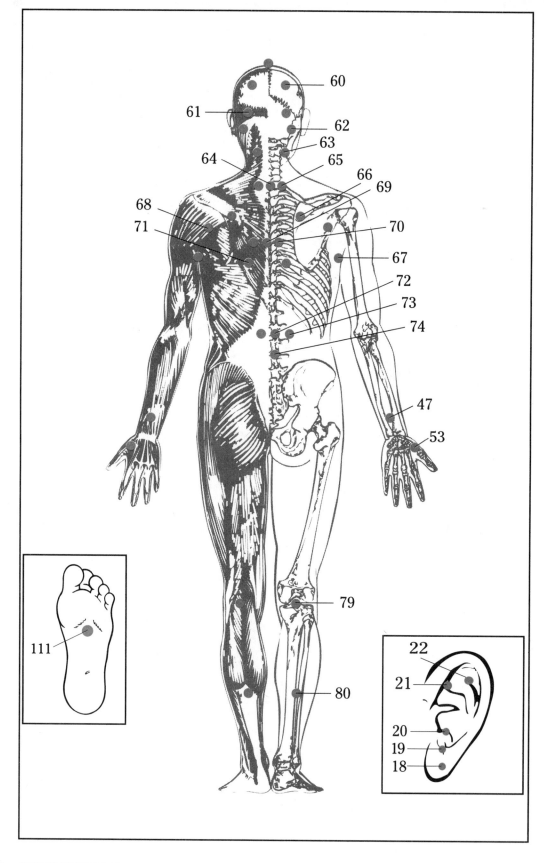

CHAPTER 2

Locations and Common Usages of the Acupressure Points.

Locations of the acupressure points and their common uses in the human body according to Traditional Chinese Medical principles.

See Charts on pages 13 and 14 for Point Locations

Order of the Points Are Given From Head to Toe

Information on page 196 will help you to find the anatomical location of the points

1. GV 20
Location: Center of the top of the head.
Used for: Headache on the top of the head, dizziness, insomnia, poor memory, hot flashes, epilepsy, mental disorders, good for memory and concentration, ringing in the ears, blurred vision, nasal obstruction, low energy, prolapse of the rectum.

2. GV 24
Location: On the midline, at the junction of the forehead and the hairline.
Used for: Frontal headaches, pressure headaches, anxiety, palpitation, insomnia, vertigo, blocked sinuses, failing memory.

3. ST 8
Location: At the corner of the forehead at the junction of the forehead and hairline.
Used for: Migraine headaches, blurred vision, common cold.

4. GB 14
Location: On the forehead, 1 body inch directly above the midpoint of the eyebrow.
Used for: Headache in the frontal area, pain in and above the eyes, twitching of the eyelids, drooping of the eyelids, glaucoma.

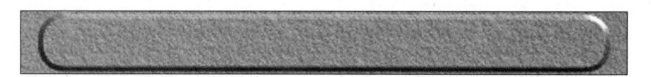

5. Yin Tang

Location: Midway between the medial end of the two eyebrows.

Used for: Frontal headache, hyperactivity, ADHD, cannot stop thinking, electro-magnetic energy imbalances, jet lag, to control addictions to food, drug, alcohol, smoking etc., to improve psychic ability, reduce mental fog, to improve memory and mental clarity, face lift point, tearing of the eyes.

6. GB 1

Location: Lateral to outer canthus, in the depression on the lateral side of the orbit.

Used for: Migraine headaches, failing vision, redness of the eye, lacrimation, glaucoma, foggy vision, cataract, face lift point.

7. Tai Yang

Location: In the depression about 1 inch posterior to the midpoint between the lateral end of the eyebrow and the outer canthus.

Used for: Headache, eye disease, deviation of the eye, deviation of the mouth, pain in the eye.

8. SI 19.

Location: Anterior to the tragus and posterior to the condyloid process of the mandible, in the depression formed when the mouth is open.

Used for: Deafness, tinnitus, ear infection, toothache, T.M.J. pain.

9. SI 18

Location: Directly below the outer canthus, in the depression on the lower border of zygoma.

Used for: Facial paralysis, twitching of the eyelids, pain in the face, toothache, swelling of the cheeks, discoloration of the sclera.

10. GB 2

Location: Anterior to the intertragic notch, at the posterior border of the condyloid process of the mandible.

Used for: Deafness, tinnitus, toothache, T.M.J. pain, facial paralysis.

11. St 7

Location: At the lower border of the zygomatic arch, in the depression anterior to the condyloid process of the mandible when the mouth is closed.

Used for: Deafness, tinnitus, ear infection, tooth ache, facial paralysis, pain in the face, T.M.J. pain.

12. UB 2

Location: On the medial end of the eyebrow, above the inner canthus.

Used for: Headache, blurred vision, failing vision, pain in the supraorbital region,

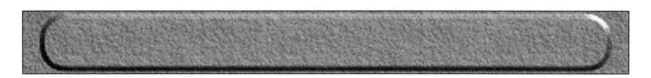

tearing of the eyes, redness of the eyes, swollen eye, pain in the eye, twitching of the eyelids, glaucoma.

13. St 2
Location: In the depression at the infra-orbital foramen.
Used for: Redness and pain of the eye, facial paralysis and pain, twitching eyelids, near sightedness, far sightedness, headaches, vertigo, face-lift point.

14. LI 20:
Location: At the level of the midpoint of the lateral border of the nostril.
Used for: Blockages of the maxillary sinuses, sinus headaches, upper respiratory problems, Common colds, nasal blockages, shortness of breath, face-lift point.

15. GV 26
Location: Below the nose, a little above the midpoint of the philtrum.
Used for: Revival point from cardiac and respiratory arrest, mental disorders, epilepsy, convulsions, coma, facial paralysis, swelling of the face, low vitality, lockjaw, diabetes, fainting spells, chest pains, heart attacks, heat stroke, middle and lower back aches, spasms of the lower back, face lift point.

16. St 4
Location: Lateral to the corner of the mouth.
Used for: Deviation of the mouth, Salivation, Twitching of the eyelid, mutism, myopia, facial palsy, to reduce fat in the thigh.

17. CV 24
Location: In the depression in the center of the mentolabial groove.
Used for: Facial paralysis, facial swelling, swelling in the lower gums, toothache, salivation, drooling.

18. Ear-Eye point (Vision clear point).
Location: In the center of the lobule.
Used for: Poor vision, eye diseases.

19. Ear-Headache (Headache control point).
Location: Below the intertragic notch.
Used for: Migraine headaches.

20. Ear-Asthma (Asthma control point).
Location: At apex of antitragus.
Used for: Asthma, bronchitis, shortness of breath.

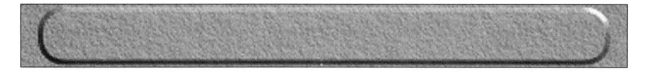

21. Sympathetic (Sweat control point).

Location: At the junction of inferior and medial part of antihelix crus.

Used for: Hyperacidity, extreme nervousness, butterfly sensation in the stomach, excessive perspiration, perspiration of the palm, sole, choking while you talk to strangers, stage fright, heart palpitation, phobia and fear of darkness, strangers etc.

22. Ear-Shenmen

Location: At the bifurcating point of upper and lower arms of the triangular fossa, slightly to the lateral side.

Used for: Stop smoking, stop overeating, calm mind, remove nervousness, pre-interview point, pre-exam point for the student, to prevent pre-nuptial jitters.

23. GB 21

Location: At the highest point of the shoulder.

Used for: Neck rigidity, pain in the shoulder, pain in the back, mastitis, arthritis of the hand and arm, to increase the bust size in women, prevent sagging breast.

24. Thymus point

Location: Beginning from the lower border of the supraclavicular fossa and extends to the upper border of the xyphoid process of the sternum.

Used for: Immune disorders, AIDS, low immunity, cancer, Epstein-barr virus diseases, frequent colds, frequent viral infections, constant allergic reactions, long term sickness, chronic fatigue syndrome, blood disorders, leukemia, spleen disorders, platelet imbalance, immature blood cell production, bone marrow diseases. Massage the entire sternal area (thymus gland) 2-3 minutes two- three times daily.

25. Lu 1

Location: In the depression below the acromial extremity of the clavicle, 8 finger breadths lateral to the midline.

Used for: Shortness of breath, upper respiratory disorders, cough, asthma, pain in the chest, pain in the shoulder and back, fullness in the chest, bronchitis, pneumonia, postnasal drip.

26. St 16

Location: In the 3rd intercostal space, 4 body inches lateral to the CV meridian.

Used for: Fullness in the chest, pain in the chest, pain in the hypochondrium, cough, asthma, mastitis, lactation deficiency.

27. CV 17

Location: On the midline of the breastbone, between the nipples, level with the 4th intercostal space.

Used for: Asthma, poor energy circulation, hiccup, pain in the chest, lactation deficiency, point to balance the energy.

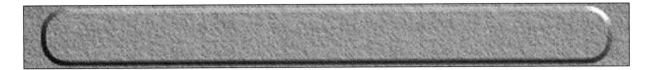

28. CV 14

Location: On the midline of the abdomen, 6 body inches above the umbilicus.

Used for: Pain in the cardiac region and the chest, nausea, acid regurgitation, difficulty in swallowing, vomiting, mental disorders, epilepsy, palpitation.

29. Kid 27

Location: In the depression below the collar bone next to the breast bone on both sides.

Used for: Anxiety, panic attacks, hiccups, cough, sore throat, balance the energy.

30. Sp 21

Location: On the mid-axillary line, 6 body inches below the axilla.

Used for: Pain in the chest, in the hypochondriac region, asthma, fibromyalgia, general body ache and general weakness.

31. CV 12

Location: On the midline of the abdomen, 5 finger breadths above the umbilicus.

Used for: Acute abdominal pain, pain due to overeating, gastric pain, sour stomach, belching, regurgitation, vomiting, diarrhea, dysentery, distention of the abdomen due to flatulence, hiatal hernia.

32. NAET Spleen point

Location: On the left side, 2 body inches lateral to CV12, on the lower border of the rib cage.

Used for: Hormone imbalances in male or female, some blood disorders, low platelet count, low white blood cell count, low red blood cell count, leukemia, imbalances in the weight (weight gain).

33. NAET Pancreas point

Location: On the left side, 1 body inch lateral to NAET Spleen point, on the lower border of the rib cage.

Used for: Hypoglycemia, diabetes, sugar craving, poor digestion of sugar, heart burns and bloating after eating sugar and starches.

34. NAET Liver point

Location: On the right side, 2 body inches lateral to CV12, on the lower border of the rib cage.

Used for: Vomiting, abdominal bloating, diarrhea, indigestion, pain in the hypochondriac area.

35. NAET Gall bladder point

Location: On the right side, 1 inch lateral to NAET Liver point, on the lower border of the rib cage.

Used for: One sided migraine headaches, frontal headache, blurred vision, hay-fever, twitching of the eyelids, twitching of any part of the body, nasal obstruction, red and painful eyes, epilepsy, fat intolerance, clay colored stool, gall stone pain.

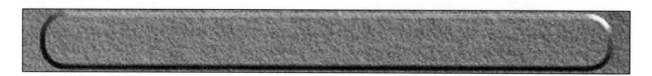

36. CV 8
Location: In the center of the umbilicus.
Used for: Abdominal pain, unchecked diarrhea, abdominal distention, flatulence, prolapse of the rectum.

37. Kid 16
Location: 0.5 body inch lateral to the umbilicus.
Used for: Abdominal pain, abdominal distention, vomiting, constipation, diarrhea.

38. St 25
Location: 3 body inches lateral (to the side) to the center of the umbilicus.
Used for: Abdominal pain, diarrhea, dysentery, constipation, gurgling sound in the abdomen due to flatus, abdominal bloating, fullness, pain around the umbilicus, water retention in the abdomen, irregular menstruation, premenstrual disorders (PMS).

39. CV 6 (General Balancing point).
Location: On the midline of the abdomen, two finger breadths below the umbilicus.
Used for: Balance the energy, abdominal pain, nocturnal emission, impotence, uterine bleeding, irregular menstruation, hernia, asthma, abdominal pain, incontinence of urine, diarrhea, constipation, abdominal distention, edema.

40. CV 4
Location: On the midline of the abdomen, 3 body inches below the umbilicus.
Used for: Enuresis, nocturnal emission, frequent urination, retention of urine, hernia, irregular menstruation, dysmenorrhea, uterine bleeding, postpartum hemorrhage, lower abdominal pain, indigestion, diarrhea, prolapse of the rectum.

41. NAET Bladder point
Location: 3 body inches below CV 8 and 4 body inches lateral on the right.
Used for: Abdominal pain, difficulty in urinating.

42. NAET large intestine point
Location: 3 body inches below CV 8 and 4 body inches lateral on the left.
Used for: Constipation, parasites, lower abdominal pain, flatulence, Abdominal bloating, indigestion.

42B. LI 13
Location: Superior to the lateral epicondyle of the humerus.
Used for: Pain in the lateral aspect of the upper arm, prevent sleeping (massage this point clockwise to keep awake).

43. NAET Kidney point
Location: 9 body inches below the axilla in the mid axillary line.
Used for: Flatulence, diarrhea, abdominal bloating, pain in the lower back.

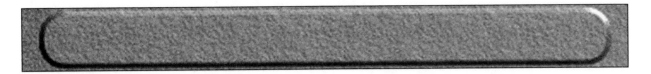

44. LI 11
Location: When the elbow is flexed, it is at the end of the elbow crease.
Used for: Food allergy, hives, vomiting, diarrhea, dysentery, fever, sore throat, pain in the elbow and arm, tennis elbow, to balance the energy in cancer patients.

45. Lu 5
Location: On the cubital crease, on the radial side of the tendon of m. biceps brachii.
Used for: Dry cough, wet cough, fever, asthma, water retention in the lungs, sore throat, chest congestion, pain in the elbow and arm, mastitis.

46. Pc 6
Location: Three finger breadths above the wrist crease on the palmar side.
Used for: Palpitation, vomiting, mental disorders, chest pains-emotional and physical, nausea, to decrease appetite, to calm down, decrease panic attacks, to stop smoking, addictions to alcohol, food and drugs, poor memory, to promote yawning, side effects of radiation and chemotherapy in cancer patients.

47. TH 5
Location: Three finger breadths above wrist crease on the dorsal side.
Used for: Headaches, pain in the cheek, jaw, TMJ problems, deafness, ringing in the ears, sensation of plugged ear, earache, pain behind the ear, pain in the hand, arthritis of the hands, hand tremor, to regulate abnormal heat sensation.

48. Ht.5
Location: 1 body inch above the wrist crease on the ulnar side.
Used for: Palpitation, dizziness, blurred vision, sore throat, hoarseness of voice, stiffness of the tongue, nervousness, pain in the wrist and arm.

49. Ht 7
Location: Medial side (ulnar) of the transverse crease of the wrist.
Used for: Chest pain, night sweat, spontaneous sweating, stage fright, phobias, nervousness (massage this point before interviews, speeches, wedding, exams, flying etc.) irritability, mental disorders, poor memory, promote mental clarity, promote retention of knowledge in the brain (good for students to massage this point five minutes before beginning study to prepare for exams etc,), chest palpitation, insomnia, nightmares, excessive dreaming, to mend broken heart, emotional stagnation, unable to cry, side effects of radiation and chemotherapy in cancer patients.

50. Lu 7
Location: Superior to the styloid process of the radius, 1.5 body inch above the transverse crease of the wrist.
Used for: Headache, migraine, neck rigidity, cough, asthma, sore throat, facial paralysis, toothache, pain and weakness of the wrist.

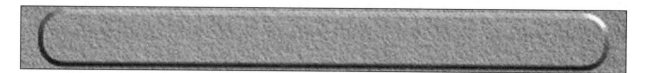

51. Lu 9

Location: Distal to the styloid process of the radius, at the radial side of the wrist crease.

Used for: Poor circulation, arterial sclerosis, Headache, migraine, neck rigidity, cough, asthma, sore throat, facial paralysis, toothache, pain and weakness of the wrist, blood disorder.

52. SI 4

Location: On the ulnar side of the palm, in the depression between the base of the fifth metacarpal bone and triquetral bone.

Used for: Fever without sweating, stiff neck, pain in the wrist, depression, phobias.

53. LI 4

Location: Midway between the thumb and index finger approximately one body inch above the web.

Used for: Headache, red eye, pain in the eye, nose bleed, toothache, sore throat, facial swelling, fever, abdominal pain, constipation, delayed menstrual cycles, absence of menstruation in fertile women without pregnancy, PMS, delayed labor, to balance the energy in the body, side effects of radiation and chemotherapy in cancer patients.

54. SI 3

Location: When a loose fist is made, this point is close to the head of the 5th metacarpal bone on the ulnar side.

Used for: Headache, stiff neck, intracranial pressure increase, glaucoma, weakness of the eye muscles, pain in the eyes, red eyes, pressure in the eyes, deafness, ringing in the ears, fever, weakness of the arm muscles, twitching of the elbow, arm and fingers, spasms of the upper back muscles, upper backache, epilepsy, night sweating.

55. Lu 11

Location: On the radial side of the thumb, posterior to the corner of the nail.

Used for: Cough, asthma, sore throat, laryngitis, nosebleed, mental fog, irritability, loss of consciousness.

56. LI 1

Location: On the radial side of the index finger, at the corner of the nail.

Used for: Great revival point, toothache, sore throat, swelling of the submandibular region, numbness of the fingers, fainting, loss of consciousness, regulate vital energy.

57. LI 2

Location: On the radial side of the index finger, distal to the metacarpo-phalangeal joint.

Used for: Toothache, blurred vision, nosebleed, sore throat, pain in the lower abdomen.

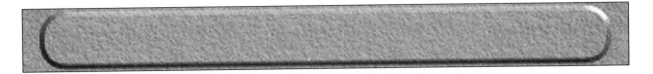

58. PC 9
Location: In the center of the tip of the middle finger.
Used for: Revival point, cardiac pain, irritability, loss of consciousness, heat stroke, febrile diseases, stiffness of the tongue, unusually warm palms and soles, fainting, poor memory, shortness of breath.

59. Ht 9
Location: On the radial side of the little finger, at the corner of the nail.
Used for: Cardiac pain, heart palpitation, pain in the chest and hypochondriac region, poor memory, fainting, mental disorders, loss of consciousness, shortness of breath.

60. GB 19
Location: Directly above GB 20, on the lateral side of the external occipital protuberance.
Used for: Headache, Stiffness of the neck, vertigo, painful eyes, tinnitus, epilepsy.

61. GB 12
Location: In the depression below the mastoid process.
Used for: Headache, insomnia, pain and stiffness of the neck, swelling of the cheek, toothache, facial paralysis, shortness of breath, great revival point from respiratory arrest.

62. Anmian
Location: Approximately 1 body inch anterior to GB 20.
Used for: Insomnia, vertigo, headache, palpitation, manic disorder, hyperactivity, mental irritability.

63. GB 20
Location: In the back of the neck, in the depression below the occipital bone.
Used for: Occipital headache, dizziness, pain and stiffness of the neck, pain in the shoulder, fever, common cold, whiplash, hypertension, weakness of the whole body.

64. GV 14
Location: Below the spinous process of the seventh cervical vertebra, approximately at the level of the shoulders.
Used for: Neck pains, stiffness, fever, epilepsy, cough, asthma, common cold, upper backache.

65. Dingchuan
Location: 0.5 body inch lateral to Cervical vertebra no. 7, below the prominent vertebra.
Used for: Asthma, cough, neck rigidity, pain in the shoulder and back.

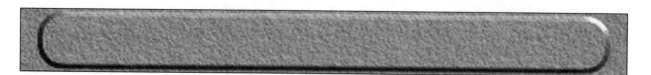

66. UB 43

Location: 4 finger breadths lateral to the spinous process of the 4th thoracic vertebra.

Used for: Cough, asthma, blood in the sputum, night sweating, tuberculosis, poor memory, indigestion, emphysema, immune deficiency disorders, cancer, chronic fatigue syndrome, low energy.

67. SI 9

Location: Posterior and inferior to the shoulder joint, directly above the posterior end of the axillary fold.

Used for: Pain in the scapular region, pain in the shoulder.

68. SI 10

Location: When the arm is adducted, the point is directly above SI 9, in the depression inferior to the scapular spine.

Used for: Pain in the shoulder, upper backache, frozen shoulder, weakness of the shoulder.

69. GV 11

Location: Below the spinous process of the 5th thoracic vertebra.

Used for: Poor memory, anxiety, palpitation, cardiac pain, pain and stiffness of the back, cough.

70. UB 15

Location: 1.5 body inch lateral to the lower border of the spinous process of the 5th thoracic vertebra.

Used for: Epilepsy, panic attack, palpitation, forgetfulness, irritability, cough, stage fright, depression, unhappy disposition, grumpy nature, never happy with anything, attitude problem.

71. UB 20.

Location: 3 finger breadths lateral to the spinous process of the 11th thoracic vertebra.

Used for: Abdominal bloating, vomiting, diarrhea, dysentery, indigestion, swelling in the abdomen, food allergy, pain in the mid-back.

72. GV 4

Location: Below the spinous process of the second lumbar vertebra.

Used for: Stiffness of the back, lumbago, impotence, nocturnal emission, irregular menstruation, diarrhea, indigestion, leukorrhea.

73. UB 23

Location: 3 finger breadths lateral to the lower border of the spinous process of the

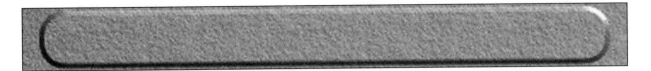

2nd lumbar vertebra.

Used for: Impotence, deafness, male disorders, low energy, sexual dysfunction in men, weakness in of the knee, blurred vision, ringing in the ears, irregular menstruation.

74. GV 3

Location: Below the spinous process of the fourth lumbar vertebra, level with the iliac crest.

Used for: Irregular menstruation, nocturnal emission, impotence, pain in the lumbosacral region, muscular atrophy, motor impairment, numbness and pain of the lower extremities.

75. Sp 10

Location: When the knee is flexed, 3 finger breadths above the superior border of the patella, on the medial side of the thigh. Feel for pain or tenderness at the spot.

Used for: Uterine bleeding, irregular menstruation, painful menstrual periods, premenstrual symptoms, absence of periods in fertile women without pregnancy, skin disorders, eczema, hives, sores in the mouth, cold sores, diabetes, sea food poisoning, any blood poisoning, acne, boils, carbuncles, furuncles etc. on the skin, kidney infection, bladder infection, septicemia, anywhere in the body, AIDS, immune deficiency disorders, herpes simplex, herpes zoster (shingles), decreased white blood cells in the blood, blood diseases, leukemia, cancer of any type, Hodgkin's disease, thyroid disorders, pain in the knee, pain in the medial part of the thigh.

76. UB 39

Location: Lateral to the midpoint of the transverse crease of the popliteal fossa.

Used for: Pain and stiffness of the lower back, lower abdominal distention, diabetes, hot palms and soles, cramps in the leg and foot, fever, abnormal sensation, dysuria, incontinence of urine.

77. Kid 10

Location: When the knee is flexed, the point is on the medial side of the popliteal fossa, between the tendons of m. semitendinosus and semimembranosus, level with UB 40.

Used for: Impotence, hernia, uterine bleeding, pain in the knee, mental disorders, brain fog, hair loss.

78. Liv 8

Location: On the medial side of the knee joint, posterior to the medial condyle of the tibia.

Used for: Lower abdominal pain, hiatal hernia, pain in the extremities, pain all over the body, dysuria, pruritus, manic disorders, pain in the external genitalia, arthritis of the knee, low sperm count, infertility in male or female, sexual dysfunction in

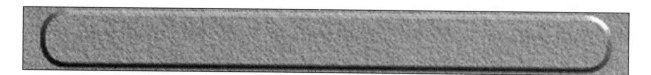

male or female, PMS, Psoriasis, skin problems, to produce sweat, insomnia, depression, anxiety attacks, venereal diseases.

79. UB 40
Location: Midpoint of the transverse crease of the popliteal fossa, between the tendons of muscle biceps femoris and muscle semitendinosus.
Used for: Low back pain, abdominal pain, vomiting, diarrhea, viral infection, bacterial infection, arthritis, fever, falling hair, falling eyebrow, pain in the lower extremities, sciatic neuralgia.

80. UB 57
Location: Directly below the belly of muscle gastrocnemius.
Used for: Cramps in the legs, varicose veins, hemorrhoids, constipation, sagging calf muscles, leg pains, low backache, poor circulation in the legs.

81. Sp 9
Location: On the lower border of the medial condyle of the knee bone (tibia), in the depression between the posterior border of the tibia and gastrocnemius muscle.
Used for: Abdominal distention, edema, water retention, incontinence of urine, difficulty urinating, not producing enough urine, kidney not able to filter enough urine, pain of the external genitalia, insomnia, painful intercourse, low libido in male or female.

82. Sp 8
Location: 3 body inches below Sp 9, on the medial border of the tibia.
Used for: Anorexia, bulimia, neurotic vomiting, abdominal distention, dysentery, severe uterine bleeding, severe uterine cramps, post partum hemorrhage, impotency, abdominal pain, diarrhea, edema, difficulty in urination, side effects of radiation and chemotherapy in cancer patients.

83. St 36
Location: Four finger breadths below the eye of the patella, one finger breadth lateral from the anterior crest of the tibia.
Used for: "Long life point", balancing point, to boost up energy, knee pain, gastric pain, vomiting, abdominal distention, diarrhea, constipation, dizziness, mental fog, mental disorders, schizophrenia, arterial sclerosis, poor digestion especially of proteins and carbohydrates, diabetes, breast abscess, mastitis, pain and swelling in the breast, side effects of radiation and chemotherapy in cancer patients.

84. Lanwei
Location: The tender spot about 2 body inches below St 36.
Used for: Acute and chronic appendicitis, indigestion, abdominal pains, abdominal spasms, poor peristalsis, incontinence of the bowel and bladder, paralysis of the lower extremities.

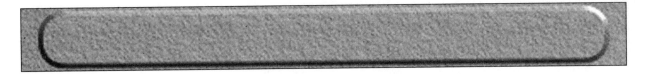

85. GB 34

Location: In the depression anterior and inferior to the head of the fibula.

Used for: Muscular atrophy, motor impairment, numbness and pain of the lower extremities, pain and swelling of the knee, pain in the hypochondriac region, bitter taste in the mouth, vomiting, weak muscles and tendons, pain in the body, tendon and muscular pains.

86. Dannang

Location: The tender spot about 2 body inches below GB 34.

Used for: Acute and chronic gall bladder pains, gall stones, muscular atrophy, numbness of the lower extremities, amoebiasis, liver flukes, parasites in the bile ducts.

87. St 37

Location: 8 Finger breadths (6 body inch) below the lateral eye of the patella, on the line connecting the eye of the patella and the external malleolus.

Used for: Abdominal bloating, severe constipation, diarrhea, dysentery, appendicitis, cramps in the lower abdomen, knee pain, colitis, irritable bowels, chrohn's disease, diverticulitis.

88. St 38

Location: 2 body inches below St 37, one finger-breadth from the anterior crest of the tibia.

Used for: Pain in the leg, numbness, soreness and pain of the knee and leg, weakness and motor impairment of the foot, pain and motor impairment of the shoulder, cramps in the leg, and abdominal pain, irritable bowels, chrohn's disease, diverticulitis.

89. St 39

Location: 3 body inches below St 37.

Used for: Lower abdominal pain, pain in the testes, mastitis, pain, numbness or paralysis of the lower limbs, irritable bowels, chrohn's disease, diverticulitis.

90. St 40

Location: 8 finger breadths above the lateral malleolus, two finger breadths lateral to the anterior crest of the tibia.

Used for: Water retention, phlegm anywhere in the body, chest pain, asthma, excessive sputum, abscesses in the internal organs, sore throat, pain of the lower leg, headaches, dizziness, mental disorders, manic disorders, schizophrenia, depression, epilepsy.

91. GB 37

Location: 5 body inches above the tip of the lateral malleolus, on the anterior border of the fibula.

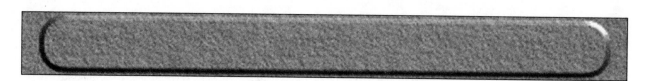

Used for: Pain in the knee, muscular atrophy, motor impairment and pain of the lower extremities, blurred vision, eye infections, vision problems due to food allergies, sty in the eye, watery eyes, puffy eyelids, itchy eyes, night blindness, pain in the breast.

92. GB39

Location: 3 body inches above the tip of the external malleolus, in the depression between the posterior border of the fibula and the tendons of m.peroneus longus and brevis.

Used for: Weakness of the limbs, stiff neck, bloating of the abdomen, pain in the hypochondriac region, muscular atrophy of the limbs, spasm and cramps of the legs, tired eyes, vision problems.

93. Kid 9

Location: At the lower end of the muscle gastrocnemius in the medial aspect, 7 finger breadths above the tip of the medial malleolus.

Used for: Pain in the medial aspect of the leg, poor water metabolism, water retention, blood poisoning, help with kidney filtration, high creatinine in the blood, high urea nitrogen, high sodium intake, high blood pressure, venereal diseases, syphilis, chemical toxemia, mental fog, poor memory, manic disorders.

94. Kid 7

Location: 3 finger breadths directly above kidney 3, on the anterior border of the tendo-calcaneus.

Used for: Improves yang energy in older people. Low backache, low energy, abdominal pain, distention, edema, swelling of the legs, weakness of the foot, paralysis of the foot, night sweating, spontaneous sweating, muscular atrophy, connective tissue disorders, myelitis, multiple sclerosis, hemorrhoids.

95. Liv 5

Location: 7 finger breadths above the tip of the medial malleolus on the medial border of tibia.

Used for: Chemical and environmental toxicity, chronic fatigue syndrome, immune deficiency disorders, irregular menstruation, PMS, fibromyalgia, dysuria, low energy, retention of urine, side effects of radiation and chemotherapy in cancer patients.

96. Sp 6

Location: 4 finger breadths directly above the tip of the medial malleolus.

Used for: Balancing point, abdominal distention, loose stools with undigested food, irregular menstruation, uterine bleeding, amenorrhea, clinical depression, immune deficiency disorders, chronic fatigue, impotence, low sperm, sterility in men and women, regulate hormone function, low sexual desire in men and women, pain in the external genitalia, warts, hemorrhoids, varicose veins, insomnia, PMS, hot flashes, cold limbs, side effects of radiation and chemotherapy in cancer patients.

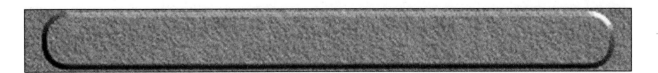

97. St 41

Location: At the junction of the dorsum of foot and the leg, between the tendons of m. extensor digitorum longus and halluces longus, approximately at the level of the tip of the external malleolus.

Used for: Edema of the head, edema of the face, dizziness, vertigo, abdominal distention, constipation, clinical depression, rheumatism, ringing in the ear, headaches.

98. Kid 3

Location: In the depression between the medial malleolus and tendo- calcaneus, level with the tip of the medial malleolus.

Used for: Balancing point, sore throat, toothache, deafness, hemoptysis, asthma, insomnia, impotence, frequency of urination, lower backache, swollen gums, palpitations, fear, emotions, anxiety attacks, vomiting, cold sores. "Ever Young point" to remove the age lines, to reduce the sensation of excessive heat or cold, side effects of radiation and chemotherapy in cancer patients.

99. UB 60

Location: In the depression between the external malleolus and tendo calcaneus.

Used for: Low backache, sciatica, radiculitis, numbness, headache, neck rigidity, blurred vision, backache, pain in the heel, epilepsy, fever, nosebleed.

100. Kid 6

Location: 1 body inch below the medial malleolus.

Used for: Irregular menstruation, PMS, prolapse of the uterus, pruritus vulvae, frequency of urination, epilepsy, insomnia, sore throat, increase psychic ability, impotence, male sexual problems.

101. Sp 4

Location: In the depression distal and inferior to the lower aspect of the 1st metatarsal bone.

Used for: Colitis, diverticulitis, Crohn's disease, gastric pain, vomiting, sour stomach, immune deficiency disorders, chronic fatigue, cancer of the stomach, inflammation of the stomach, gastric ulcers, internal hemorrhage, ascites, pleurisy, epilepsy, arthritis, depression, anxiety attacks, irritable bowls.

102. Liv 3

Location: In the depression distal to the junction of the 1st and 2nd metatarsal bones.

Used for: Balancing point, low energy, hypertension, uterine bleeding, PMS, retention of urine, abdominal distention, fever, diarrhea, headache, chemical toxicity, anger, epilepsy, bleeding from the stomach, bleeding from the eyes, mouth, mucus membrane, stroke, infantile convulsion, poor circulation.

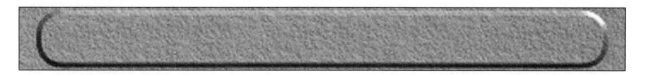

103. St 44

Location: Proximal to the web between the 2nd and 3rd toes, in the depression distal and lateral to the 2nd metatarso-digital joint.

Used for: Toothache, frontal headache, nasal congestion, dental anaesthesia, laryngitis, pain during menstrual periods, nose bleed, abdominal pain, food retention, fever.

104. GB 41

Location: In the depression distal to the junction of the fourth and fifth metatarsal bones, on the lateral side of the tendon of m. extensor digiti minimi of the foot.

Used for: Headache, vertigo, pain in the outer canthus, pain in the upper abdomen, pain in the breast, irregular menstruation, pain and swelling of the dorsum of the foot, neuroma, spasm of the foot and toe.

105. UB 66

Location: In the depression anterior and inferior to the 5th metatarso-phalangeal joint.

Used for: Mental disorders, headache, stiff neck, blurred vision, backache, pain in the legs.

106. Sp 1

Location: On the medial side of the great toe, 0.1 body inch posterior to the corner of the nail.

Used for: Bloody stool, severe uterine bleeding, dream disturbed sleep, mental disorders, convulsions, diarrhea, dysentery, PMS, fear in children, fatigue, temper tantrum in children, hyperactivity, arthritis, anxiety attacks.

107. Liv 1

Location: On the lateral side of the great toe, between the lateral corner of the nail and the interphalangeal joint.

Used for: Hernia, uterine bleeding, prolapse of the uterus, epilepsy, difficulty in urination, incontinence of urine, pain in the groin.

108. St 45

Location: On the lateral side of the 2nd toe, 0.1 body inch posterior to the corner of the nail.

Used for: Facial swelling, deviation of the mouth, facial palsy, nose bleed, toothache, sore throat, hoarse voice, abdominal distention, coldness in the leg and foot, fever, dream-disturbed sleep, nightmares, food poisoning, abdominal pains due to over eating.

109. GB 44

Location: On the lateral side of the fourth toe, about 0.1 body inch posterior to the corner of the nail.

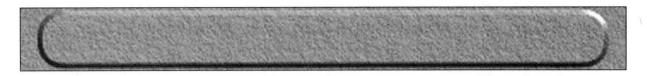

Used for: Migraine, deafness, ringing in the ears, eye troubles, like poor vision, blurred vision, infection, red eye, fever, dream disturbed sleep.

110. UB 67

Location: On the lateral side of the small toe, about 0.1 body inch posterior to the corner of the nail.

Used for: Headache, nasal obstruction, nose bleed, eye problems, eye infection, poor vision, blurred vision, difficult labor, backache, pain in the lower extremities, heat sensation in the sole.

111. Kid 1

Location: In the depression appearing on the sole when the foot is in plantar flexion, approximately at the junction of the anterior and middle third of the sole.

Used for: Revival point, drowning, heart problem, sterility, muscular dystrophy, pain in the vertex, dizziness, blurred vision, sore throat, dryness of the tongue, aphonia, fevers.

CHAPTER 3

Acupressure
Guidelines

The information in this book will provide you with temporary help to alleviate your health problems and emergencies. If your problems persist, please see a physican.

Any of the following health disorders may be arising from immediate allergies or an accumulation of various reactions over a period of time. It is for the patient's benefit to consult with a NAET practitioner to evaluate his/her condition. When you find your allergies and eliminate them permanently through NAET, you may be able to be free of these unpleasant health conditions forever. In some cases it may be easy to eliminate the problem in just a few treatments. Often however, your problems may be the result of a number of allergens reacting in your body over a long period of time. For the chronically ill patients, several NAET treatments may be required before they can get maximum benefits. If you have a weak immune system, and suffer from any of the health disorders mentioned in this book, you may benefit from stimulating (massaging) the acupressure points related to the disorders described in this book.

Readers who are NAET patients, please remember to follow the instructions in the NAET Guide book.

ALWAYS TREAT THE "BASIC TEN" ALLERGIES FIRST.

The Basic ten are:

1. Egg mix (Egg yolk, egg white, chicken, animal proteins).

2. Calcium mix (3 calcium groups, cow's milk and goat's milk).

3. Vitamin C mix (3 vitamin C group, fruits, and vegetables).

4. B complex (17 B complex vitamins).

5. Sugar mix (13 sugars).

6. Iron mix (3 iron groups, 3 red meats).

7. Vitamin A mix (Fish, shell fish, salmon, beta carotene, vit. A).

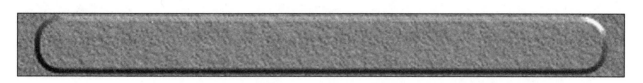

8. Mineral mix (63 trace minerals and essential minerals).

9. Salt mix (Sodium chloride).

10. Grain mix (Wheat, corn, rice, barley, oats, millet).

A few commonly seen health conditions and usual allergens that cause these problems have been given in the next few pages.

In any acute type of problem, where the problem suddenly occurs, and the person is suffering from pain or discomfort continuously for 24 - 48 hours, always look for something the person drank (e.g. milk, juice, water), ate (eg. apple, donut, cracker), touched (e.g. cosmetics, clothes, work materials), breathed (e.g. perfume, grass pollens, cat litter), or an emotionally strained incident (e.g. unpleasant confrontation with a person, loss of a loved one, loss of job, property damage, spiritual trauma). NOTHING ACUTE IN NATURE TAKES PLACE IN OUR BODY WITHOUT HAVING ONE OF THESE CAUSES.

1. ABDOMINAL BLOATING

COMMONLY SEEN ALLERGENS: Allergy to any food or drink you had within 24-48 hours, Basic ten, milk products, vitamin C, B complex, sugar, iron, cold, heat, dried beans, spices, salt, fats, turkey, grains, alcohol, acid, base, food additives, fabrics, chemicals, wood, pollens, weeds, flowers, and emotional upsets.

ACUTAP/MASSAGE POINTS: CV6(p.39), St25(p.38), LI4(p.53), St36 (p.83), St37 (p.87), Liv3(p.102), St41(p.97).

2. ABDOMINAL PAIN

COMMONLY SEEN ALLERGENS: Allergy to any food or drink you had within 24-48 hours, Basic ten, Animal fats, vegetable fats, spices, sugar, fried foods, uncooked foods, parasites, chemicals from food or environments, water chemicals, milk or milk products.

ACUTAP/MASSAGE POINTS: CV6(p.39), St36(p.83), Sp8(p.82), St 44(p.103), CV12(p.31), LI4(p.53), St25(p.38), St37(p.87), St39(p.89), GV26(p.15), Pc6(p.46).

3. ABDOMINAL PAINS DUE TO OVEREATING (Upper side of the abdomen).

COMMONLY SEEN ALLERGENS: Allergy to any food or drink you had within 24-48 hours.

ACUTAP/MASSAGE POINTS: St44(p.103), CV12(p.31), St36(p.83), St45(p.108), LI2(p.57).

4. ABDOMINAL SPASMS (Colic)

COMMONLY SEEN ALLERGENS: Allergy to any food or drink you had within 24-48 hours, milk products, juice, water, dried beans.

ACUTAP/MASSAGE POINTS: Lanwei(p.84), CV8(p.36), UB20(p.71), St44 (p.103), LI2(p.57), NAET UB(p.41), NAET LI(p.42), NAET Ut(p.40).

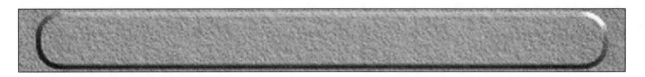

5. LOWER ABDOMINAL PAIN

COMMONLY SEEN ALLERGENS: Allergy to any food or drink you had within 24-48 hours, Basic ten, soaps, lotions, items causing low energy flow during menstrual periods (PMS) like sugar, chocolate, salt, spices, foods and drinks causing constipation, clothes around the lower abdomen like underpants, elastics, cold, sanitary napkins.

ACUTAP/MASSAGE POINTS: LI2(p.57), LI4(p.53), St37(p.87), Sp6(p.96), NAET Ut(p.40),

6. ACUTE VIRAL INFECTION

COMMONLY SEEN ALLERGENS: Allergy to any food or drink you had within 24-48 hours.

ACUTAP/MASSAGE POINTS: Sp10(p.75), Thymus(p.24), LI11 (p.44), UB40(p.79), CV12(p.31), GB20(p.63).

7 ACUTE APPENDICITIS

COMMONLY SEEN ALLERGENS: Allergy to any food or drink you had within 24-48 hours, tropical fruits, nuts, seeds, beans, fried food, cheese, milk products.

ACUTAP/MASSAGE POINTS: Lanwei(p.84), LI2(p.57), St36(p.83), St37(p.87), GV26(p.15).

8. ADHD (Attention Deficit and Hyperactive Disorder).

COMMONLY SEEN ALLERGENS: Basic ten, individual sugars, wheat, gluten, corn, tomato, peppers, food additives, food colors, refined starches, spices, parasites, bacteria, pesticides, molds, fabrics, detergents, perfumes, chemicals, hormones, crayons, paper, ink, coloring papers, school materials, books, school bags, shampoo, lipstick, nylons, trace minerals, and alcohol.

ACUTAP/MASSAGE POINTS: Yintang(p.5), Pc6(p.46), Ht7(p.49), NAET SP (p.32), NAET LIV(p.34), LI11(p.44), CV12(p.31), E-shenmen(p.22).

9. ACNE

COMMONLY SEEN ALLERGENS: Basic ten, Animal fats, vegetable fats, spices, sugar, fried foods, sugar and fat together, hormones, grains, stomach acids, digestive enzymes, yeast, candida, cosmetics, contamination of the skin by infected agents, poor digestion, emotional blockages, poor elimination and not drinking enough water.

ACUTAP/MASSAGE POINTS: Sp10(p.75), LI11(p.44), St25(p.37), St37(p.87), NAET LI(p.42).

10. ADDICTION TO FOOD, DRUGS, CAFFEINE, CHOCOLATE AND ALCOHOL

COMMONLY SEEN ALLERGENS: Basic ten, B complex, sugar, trace minerals, emotions.

ACUTAP/MASSAGE POINTS: Yintang(p.5), Pc6(p.46), Ht7(p.49), NAET Liv(p.34), ear-shenmen(p.22).

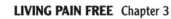

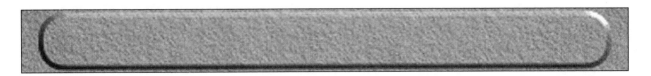

11. ANGER

COMMONLY SEEN ALLERGENS: Basic ten, protein, individual B vitamins, vitamin C, sugar, colors, food additives, wheat, corn, gluten, fats, alcohol, work materials like wood, paper, paint, formaldehyde and emotional blockages.

ACUTAP/MASSAGE POINTS: Liv3(p.102), NAET Liv(p.34), Ht7(p.49), Pc6(p.46), SI4(p.52), LI11(p.44).

12. ANGIONEUROTIC EDEMA:

COMMONLY SEEN ALLERGENS: Allergy to any food or drink you had within 24-48 hours, Basic ten, bioflavanoids, citrus fruits, physical activity like running, cycling, etc.

ACUTAP/MASSAGE POINTS: Thymus(p.24), NAET Lu(p.25), Kid9(p.93), Sp9(p.81), Pc6(p.46), LI11(p.44), CV12(p.31), GB12(p.61).

13. ANOREXIA NERVOSA

COMMONLY SEEN ALLERGENS: Basic ten, coffee, chocolate, food colors, artificial sweeteners, food additives, yeast, pesticides, emotional blockages.

ACUTAP/MASSAGE POINTS: Sp8(p.82), CV12(p.31), Pc6(p.46), Ht7(p.49), SI4(p.52).

14. ANXIETY ATTACKS

COMMONLY SEEN ALLERGENS: Allergy to any food or drink you had within 24-48 hours, Basic ten, peanut butter, nuts, vegetable oils, whiten-all, turkey, chocolate, water chemicals.

ACUTAP/MASSAGE POINTS: GV24(p.2), GV11(p.69), Liv8(p.78), Sp4(p.101), Kid3(p.98), Sp1(p.106).

15. ARTHRITIS OF THE FINGERS

COMMONLY SEEN ALLERGENS: Basic ten, Proteins, calcium, vitamin C, citrus fruits, B complex, sugar, iron, hormones, trace minerals, carbonated drinks, ice cream, cold meats, chocolate, coffee, tea, fats, spices, artificial sweeteners, turkey, pollens, weeds, flowers, wood, smoke, cigarette smoke, emotional factors, chemicals, cleaning agents, gloves, bacteria, rings, jewelry, newspaper, pens, pencils, nail polish, pesticides, formaldehyde, stomach acids, base, heat, cold, handicraft materials, plastics, computer keyboard, paints, and fabrics.

ACUTAP/MASSAGE POINTS: TH5(p.47), Pc6(p.46), Ht7(p.49).

16. ARTHRITIS OF THE HAND

COMMONLY SEEN ALLERGENS: Basic ten, proteins, calcium, vitamin C, citrus fruits, B complex, sugar, iron, hormones, trace minerals, carbonated drinks, ice cream, cold meats, chocolate, coffee, tea, fats, spices, artificial sweeteners, turkey, pollens, weeds, flowers, wood, smoke, cigarette smoke, emotional factors, chemicals, cleaning agents,

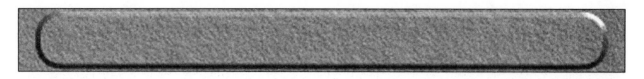

gloves, bacteria, pesticides, formaldehyde, pen, pencil, newspaper, rings, wrist watch, stomach acids, base, heat, cold, and fabrics.

ACUTAP/MASSAGE POINTS: TH5(p.47), Ht5(p.48), Pc6(p.46).

17. ARTHRITIS OF THE ELBOW

COMMONLY SEEN ALLERGENS: Basic ten, proteins, calcium, vitamin C, citrus fruits, B complex, sugar, iron, hormones, trace minerals, carbonated drinks, ice cream, cold meats, chocolate, coffee, tea, fats, spices, artificial sweeteners, turkey, wood, emotional factors, chemicals, cleaning agents, gloves, writing desk, arm rest of the car, furniture, watch, jewelry, bacteria, pesticides, formaldehyde, pen, pencil, newspaper, stomach acids, base, heat, cold, and fabrics.

ACUTAP/MASSAGE POINTS: LI11(p.44), Lu5(p.45), GB21(p.23).

18. ARTHRITIS OF THE SHOULDER

COMMONLY SEEN ALLERGENS: Basic ten, proteins, calcium, vitamin C, citrus fruits, B complex, sugar, iron, hormones, trace minerals, carbonated drinks, ice cream, cold meats, chocolate, coffee, tea, fats, spices, artificial sweeteners, turkey, emotional factors, chemicals, cleaning agents, gloves, pillow, bed sheets, bacteria, pesticides.

ACUTAP/MASSAGE POINTS: Lu1(p.25), GB21(p.23), SI9(p.67), SI10(p.68), NAET Sp(p.32).

19. ARTHRITIS OF THE WRIST

COMMONLY SEEN ALLERGENS: Basic ten, proteins, calcium, vitamin C, citrus fruits, B complex, sugar, iron, hormones, trace minerals, carbonated drinks, cold meats, fats, spices, artificial sweeteners, emotional factors, chemicals, cleaning agents, gloves, watch, jewelry, bacteria, pesticides, formaldehyde, pen, pencil, newspaper, and fabrics.

ACUTAP/MASSAGE POINTS: Ht7(p.49), TH5(p.47), Pc6(p.46), NAET Kid(p.43).

20. ARTHRITIS OF THE HIP JOINT

COMMONLY SEEN ALLERGENS: Basic ten, proteins, calcium, vitamin C, citrus fruits, B complex, sugar, iron, hormones, trace minerals, carbonated drinks, ice cream, cold meats, chocolate, coffee, tea, fats, spices, artificial sweeteners, turkey, wood, smoke, cigarette smoke, emotional factors, chemicals, water chemicals, elastics, bacteria, pesticides, formaldehyde, chair, stomach acids, base, heat, cold, and fabrics.

ACUTAP/MASSAGE POINTS: NAET Kid(p.43), CV4(p.40), Kid10(p.77), GV3(p.74), NAET UB(p.41), NAET LI(p.42), Pc6(p.46), St37(p.87).

21. ARTHRITIS OF THE KNEE

COMMONLY SEEN ALLERGENS: Basic ten, proteins, calcium, vitamin C, citrus fruits,

B complex, sugar, iron, salt, hormones, trace minerals, carbonated drinks, ice cream, cold meats, chocolate, coffee, tea, fats, spices, artificial sweeteners, turkey, emotional factors, chemicals, water chemicals, elastics, bacteria, pesticides, shoe, socks, formaldehyde, chair, stomach acids, base, heat, cold, and fabrics.

ACUTAP/MASSAGE POINTS: UB40(p.79), Sp10(p.75), UB39(p.76), Liv8(p.78), Sp9(p.81), St36(p.83), St37(p.87).

22. ARTHRITIS OF THE ANKLES AND TOES

COMMONLY SEEN ALLERGENS: Basic ten, proteins, calcium, vitamin C, citrus fruits, B complex, sugar, iron, hormones, trace minerals, carbonated drinks, ice cream, cold meats, chocolate, coffee, tea, fats, spices, artificial sweeteners, turkey, emotional factors, chemicals, water chemicals, elastics, jewelry, bacteria, pesticides, shoe, socks, formaldehyde, chair, stomach acids, base, heat, cold, and fabrics.

ACUTAP/ MASSAGE POINTS: Liv8(p.78), Sp9(p.81), UB60(p.99), Kid 3(p.98), GB41(p.104), GB39(p.92).

23. OSTEO ARTHRITIS

COMMONLY SEEN ALLERGENS: Basic ten, proteins, vitamin D, citrus fruits, B complex vitamins, sugar, calcium, sodium, phosphorus, magnesium, hormones, boron, iron, salt, stomach acid, base, digestive enzymes, potassium, wheat, corn, yeast, yogurt, whey, vegetable fats, animal fats, alcohols, chemicals, cold.

ACUTAP/MASSAGE POINTS: SI3(p.54), GV26(p.15), Sp10(p.75), St36(p.83), LI4(p.53), LI11(p.44), Liv3(p.102), Liv5(p.95), Sp6(p.96), Sp21(p.30).

24. RHEUMATOID ARTHRITIS

COMMONLY SEEN ALLERGENS: Basic ten, proteins, vitamin C products, B complex vitamins, sugar, calcium, bacteria mix, chemicals, sodium, phosphorus, magnesium, hormones, boron, iron, stomach acid, base, vitamin D, digestive enzymes, potassium, wheat, corn, yeast, yogurt, whey, vegetable fats, animal fats, alcohols, cold.

ACUTAP/MASSAGE POINTS: SI3(p.54), GV26(p.15), Sp10(p.75), Sp4(p.101), LI4(p.58), LI11(p.44), Liv3(p.102), Liv5(p.95), Sp6(p.96), Sp21(p.30).

25. LUPUS ARTHRITIS

COMMONLY SEEN ALLERGENS: Basic ten, proteins, vitamin C products, B complex vitamins, sugar, calcium, bacteria mix, chemicals, sodium, phosphorus, magnesium, hormones, boron, iron, salt, stomach acid, base, vitamin D, digestive enzymes, potassium, wheat, corn, yeast, yogurt, whey, vegetable fats, animal fats, alcohols, cold, fabric (especially cotton).

ACUTAP/MASSAGE POINTS: SI3(p.54), GV26(p.15), Sp10(p.75), Sp4(p.101), LI4(p.53), LI11(p.44), Liv3(p.102), Liv5(p.95), Sp6(p.96), Sp21(p.30).

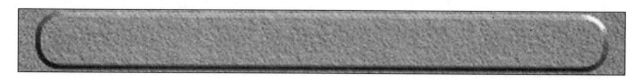

26. ASCITES

COMMONLY SEEN ALLERGENS: Basic ten, calcium, iron, water chemicals, dried beans, spices, salt, fats, turkey, food additives, parasites, emotions.

ACUTAP/MASSAGE POINTS: Sp4(p.101), Sp9(p.81), St25(p.38), St40(p.90).

27. ASTHMA

COMMONLY SEEN ALLERGENS: Allergy to any food or drink you had within 24-48 hours, Basic ten, proteins, calcium, vitamin C, fruits, B complex, sugar, carbonated drinks, chocolate, coffee, tea, fats, spices, artificial sweeteners, turkey, pollens, weeds, flowers, wood, smoke, cigarette smoke, emotional factors, chemicals, pesticides, stomach acids, base, heat, cold, humidity and fabrics.

ACUTAP/MASSAGE POINTS: Lu1(p.25), St16(p.26), CV6(p.39), Kid27(p.29), Lu11(p.55), GV14(p.64), Lu5(p.45), Lu7(p.50), UB43(p.66), St40(p.90), Kid3(p.98), CV17(p.26), E-asthma(p.20), Dingchuan(p.65).

28. BACKACHE, LOWER (Lower Backache)

COMMONLY SEEN ALLERGENS: Basic ten, calcium, iron, cold, heat, dried beans, spices, salt, fats, turkey, beds, sheets, detergents, fabrics, elastics, milk products, grains, chemicals, gelatin, chair, desk, wood, and emotions.

ACUTAP/MASSAGE POINTS: UB40(p.79), GV26(P.15), LI2(p.57), GV4(p.72), Pc6(p.46).

29. BACKACHE, MIDDLE

COMMONLY SEEN ALLERGENS: Basic ten, cold, heat, dried beans, spices, fats, turkey, potato, milk products, potato, tomato, bell pepper, gelatin, beds, sheets, detergents, fabrics, elastics, chemicals, chair, desk, wood, and emotional blockages.

ACUTAP/MASSAGE POINTS: UB20(p.71), CV12(p.31), CV14(p.28), St36(p.83), NAET Kid(p.43), NAET Sp(p.32), NAET Liv(p.34), Pc6(p.46).

30. BACKACHE, UPPER (upper backache)

COMMONLY SEEN ALLERGENS: Basic ten, iron, tomato, cold, heat, dried beans, spices, fats, turkey, milk products, grains, gelatin, name tags on the shirt, formaldehyde, beds, sheets, detergents, fabrics, chemicals, chair, desk, wood, and emotional blockages.

ACUTAP/MASSAGE POINTS: SI3(p.54), GB21(p.23), GB20(p.63), GV14(p.64), TH5(p.47).

31. BACTERIAL INFECTION

COMMONLY SEEN ALLERGENS: Allergy to any food or drink you had within 24-48 hours, Basic ten, milk, vitamin C, B complex, sugar, iron, cold, heat, dried beans, spices, salt, turkey, grains, food additives, detergents, fabrics, tap water.

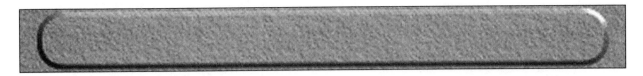

ACUTAP/MASSAGE POINTS: UB40(p.79), LI11(p.44), Sp10(p.75), Thymus(p.24).

32. BLEEDING FROM THE GUMS

COMMONLY SEEN ALLERGENS: Basic ten, cold, heat, candida or yeast infections, milk products, tooth brush, tooth paste, chemicals, citrus fruits and drinks.

ACUTAP/MASSAGE POINTS: Thumus (p.24), CU12 (p.31), NAET SP (p.32), LU 9 (p.51), SP 10 (p.75), LIV 3 (p.102).

33. BLEEDING FROM THE NOSE

COMMONLY SEEN ALLERGENS: Allergy to any food or drink you had within 24-48 hours, Basic ten, milk, vitamin C, B complex, sugar, iron, cold, heat, dried beans, vinegar, spices, salt, fats, turkey, grains, food additives, beds, sheets, detergents, fabrics, kleenex, carpets, chemicals, chair, desk, wood, pollens, weeds, flowers, paper towels, toilette paper, and emotional blockages.

ACUTAP/MASSAGE POINTS: NAET Liv(p.34), LI20(p.14), Kid3(p.98), UB60(p.97).

34. BLEEDING FROM THE EYES

COMMONLY SEEN ALLERGENS: Allergy to any food or drink you had within 24-48 hours, Basic ten, milk, vitamin C, B complex, vitamin A, fish, sugar, iron, cold, heat, wind, smog, chemical fumes.

ACUTAP/MASSAGE POINTS: Liv3(p.102), Sp10(p.75), Lu9(p.51), Thymus(P.24).

35. BLEEDING FROM THE MOUTH

COMMONLY SEEN ALLERGENS: Allergy to any food or drink you had within 24-48 hours, Basic ten, milk, vitamin C, B complex, sugar, iron, cold, heat, dried beans, vinegar, spices, salt, fats, turkey, grains, food additives, fabrics, kleenex, chemicals, and emotional blockages.

ACUTAP/MASSAGE POINTS: Liv3(p.102), Sp10(p.75), Lu9(p.51), Thymus(P.24).

36. BLEEDING FROM THE MUCOUS MEMBRANE

COMMONLY SEEN ALLERGENS: Allergy to any food or drink you had within 24-48 hours, Basic ten, milk, vitamin C, B complex, sugar, iron, cold, heat, dried beans, vinegar, spices, salt, fats, turkey, grains, food additives, fabrics, chemicals.

ACUTAP/MASSAGE POINTS: Liv3(p.102), Sp10(p.75), LU9(p.51), Thymus(P.24).

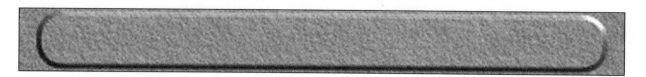

37. BLEEDING FROM THE STOMACH

COMMONLY SEEN ALLERGENS: Allergy to any food or drink you had within 24-48 hours, Basic ten, milk, vitamin C, B complex, sugar, iron, cold, heat, dried beans, vinegar, spices, salt, fats, turkey, grains, food additives, fabrics, chemicals.

ACUTAP/MASSAGE POINTS: Liv3(p.102), Sp10(p.75), Lu9(p.51), Thymus(P.24), CV12(p.31).

38. BLOOD DISORDERS

COMMONLY SEEN ALLERGENS: Allergy to any food or drink you had within 24-48 hours, Basic ten, milk, vitamin C, B complex, sugar, iron, cold, heat, dried beans, vinegar, spices, salt, fats, turkey, grains, food additives, pesticides, grasses, pollens, weeds, parasites, fabrics, chemicals.

ACUTAP/MASSAGE POINTS: Thymus(p.24), NAET Sp(p.32), Sp10(p.75), UB43(p.66), Sp8(p.82), Lu9(p.51).

39. BLOOD IN THE STOOL

COMMONLY SEEN ALLERGENS: Allergy to any food or drink you had within 24-48 hours, Basic ten, milk, vitamin C, B complex, sugar, iron, cold, heat, dried beans, vinegar, spices, salt, fats, turkey, grains, food additives, pesticides, detergents, fabrics, water chemicals, parasites.

ACUTAP/MASSAGE POINTS: Sp1(p.106), Kid16(p.37), St37(p.87), Sp4(p.101).

40. BLOOD IN THE URINE

COMMONLY SEEN ALLERGENS: Allergy to any food or drink you had within 24-48 hours, Basic ten, milk, vitamin C, B complex, sugar, iron, cold, heat, dried beans, vinegar, spices, garlic, onion, salt, fats, turkey, grains, food additives, pesticides, detergents, fabrics, water chemicals, parasites.

ACUTAP/MASSAGE POINTS: Sp10(p.75), Sp1(p.106), Kid16(p.37), CV4(p.40), UB60(p.99).

41. BLEEDING FROM THE UTERUS(excessive uterine bleeding).

COMMONLY SEEN ALLERGENS: Allergy to any food or drink you had within 24-48 hours, Basic ten, milk, vitamin C, B complex, sugar, iron, cold, heat, dried beans, vinegar, spices, garlic, onion, alfalfa, chlorophyll, salt, fats, turkey, grains, food additives, pesticides, detergents, fabrics, water chemicals, parasites, sanitary napkins, tampons.

ACUTAP/MASSAGE POINTS: Sp1(p.106), Sp8(p.82).

42. BLEEDING FROM THE RECTUM

COMMONLY SEEN ALLERGENS: Allergy to any food or drink you had within 24-48 hours,

Basic ten, milk products, vitamin C, sugar, iron, tomato, spices, fats, turkey, grains, food additives, food colors, detergents, fabrics, nylons, underpants, cotton crotches on the underpants, chemicals.

ACUTAP/MASSAGE POINTS: Sp1(p.106), Sp4(p.101), St37(p.87), Sp8(p.82).

43. HEMORRHOIDS, BLEEDING OR IRRITATION

COMMONLY SEEN ALLERGENS: Allergy to any food or drink you had within 24-48 hours, Basic ten, milk products, vitamin C, sugar, iron, tomato, spices, fats, turkey, grains, food additives, food colors, detergents, fabrics, nylons, underpants, cotton crotches on the underpants, chemicals.

ACUTAP/MASSAGE POINTS: UB57(p.80), UB60(p.99), Sp6(p.96), Sp8(p.82), Lu9(p.51), LI2(p.57).

44. BURNING FEET

COMMONLY SEEN ALLERGENS: Basic ten, vitamin C, B complex, vitamin B3, sugar, iron, cold, heat, artificial sweeteners, dried beans, spices, salt, fats, turkey, grains, alcohol, acid, base, food additives, some fabrics, socks, shoes, chemicals, wood, pollens, weeds, flowers, and emotional blockages.

ACUTAP/MASSAGE POINTS: UB60(p.99), Sp6(p.96), St36(p.83), K3(p.98), K7(p.94), Sp4(p.101).

45. BLOCKED SINUSES

COMMONLY SEEN ALLERGENS: Allergy to any food or drink you had within 24-48 hours, Basic ten, milk products, vitamin C, sugar, iron, tomato, spices, fats, turkey, grains, food additives, food colors, detergents, fabrics, nylons, underpants, cotton crotches on the underpants, chemicals.

ACUTAP/MASSAGE POINTS: LI20(p.14), Gv24(p.2), GV20(p.1), St2(p.13), UB2(p.12), GB20(p.63), LI4(p.53).

46. BLURRED VISION

COMMONLY SEEN ALLERGENS: Allergy to any food or drink you had within 24-48 hours, Basic ten, milk products, vitamin C, sugar, iron, tomato, spices, fats, turkey, grains, food additives, food colors, detergents, fabrics, nylons, underpants, cotton crotches on the underpants, chemicals.

ACUTAP/ MASSAGE POINTS: GB37(p.91), UB2(p.12), GB14(p.4), St8(p.3), GV20(p.1), GB41(p.104), NAET GB(p.35), NAET Liv(p.34), E-eye(p.18).

47. BRAIN FOG

COMMONLY SEEN ALLERGENS: Basic ten, proteins, calcium, vitamin C, citrus fruits, B complex, sugar, iron, hormones, trace minerals, carbonated drinks, ice cream, cold meats, chocolate, coffee, tea, fats, spices, artificial sweeteners, turkey, pollens, weeds,

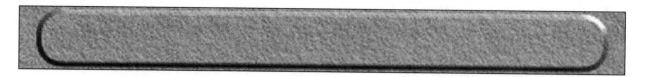

flowers, wood, smoke, cigarette smoke, emotional factors, chemicals, cleaning agents, gloves, bacteria, pesticides, formaldehyde, pen, pencil, newspaper, rings, wrist watch, stomach acids, base, heat, cold, and fabrics.

ACUTAP/MASSAGE POINTS: Kid10(p.77), Ht7(p.49), Ht9(p.59), NAET Kid(p.43), Kid7(p.94), Kid3(p.98).

48. BREAST PAIN

COMMONLY SEEN ALLERGENS: Basic ten, proteins, calcium, soybean, vitamin C, chlorophyll, citrus fruits, B complex, sugar, iron, hormones, trace minerals, potato, corn, chocolate, coffee, tea, fats, spices, artificial sweeteners, cigarette smoke, emotional factors, chemicals, cleaning agents, pesticides, formaldehyde, stomach acids, fabrics.

ACUTAP/MASSAGE POINTS: St36(p.83), Pc6(p.46), Ht7(p.49), CV12(p.31), Liv3(p.102), St16(p.26).

49. BRONCHITIS

COMMONLY SEEN ALLERGENS: Allergy to any food or drink you had couple of days before the bronchitis started. Basic ten, proteins, calcium, vitamin C, citrus fruits, B complex, sugar, iron, hormones, trace minerals, carbonated drinks, ice cream, cold meats, chocolate, coffee, tea, fats, spices, artificial sweeteners, turkey, pollens, weeds, flowers, wood, smoke, cigarette smoke, emotional factors, chemicals, cleaning agents, gloves, bacteria, pesticides, formaldehyde, pen, pencil, newspaper, rings, wrist watch, stomach acids, base, heat, cold, and fabrics.

ACUTAP/MASSAGE POINTS: E-asthma(p.20), Lu1(25), Lu7(p.50), St 40(p.90), Kid3(p.98), Lu5(p.45), thymus(p.24).

50. BULIMIA

COMMONLY SEEN ALLERGENS: Basic ten, proteins, calcium, soybean, vitamin C, citrus fruits, B complex, sugar, iron, hormones, trace minerals, potato, corn, chocolate, coffee, tea, fats, spices, artificial sweeteners, cigarette smoke, emotional factors, chemicals, cleaning agents, pesticides, formaldehyde, stomach acids, fabrics.

ACUTAP/MASSAGE POINTS: Sp8(p.82), CV12(p.31), Pc6(p.46).

51. BUTTERFLY SENSATION IN THE STOMACH OR NERVOUS STOMACH

COMMONLY SEEN ALLERGENS: Basic ten, proteins, calcium, vitamin C, B complex, sugar, iron, hormones, trace minerals, corn, chocolate, coffee, chemicals, cleaning agents, pesticides, formaldehyde, stomach acids, fabrics.

ACUTAP/MASSAGE POINTS: E-Sweat(p.21), CV14(p.28), Pc6(p.46), DU26(p.15).

52. CARDIAC ARREST AND RESPIRATORY ARREST

COMMONLY SEEN ALLERGENS: Allergy to any food, drink, chemical exposure, you had within 24-48 hours, Basic ten, alcohol, food additives, some fabrics, chemicals, pesti-

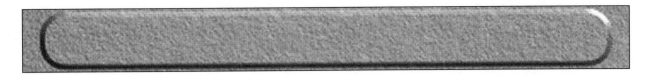

cides, emotional blockages.

ACUTAP/MASSAGE POINTS: GV26(p.15), GB12(p.61), Pc9(p.58), LI1(p.56), Ht9(p.59), Kid1(p.111), GB20(p.63), UB15(p.70), GV11(p.69).

53. CARDIAC PAIN (chest pain)

COMMONLY SEEN ALLERGENS: Allergy to any food, drink, chemical exposure, you had within 24-48 hours, basic ten, alcohol, food additives, some fabrics, chemicals, pesticides, emotional blockages.

ACUTAP/MASSAGE POINTS: GV11(p.69), Pc6(p.46), Pc9(p.58), Ht9(p.59),

54. CELIAC SPRUE

COMMONLY SEEN ALLERGENS: Basic ten, proteins, calcium, milk products, vitamin C, fruits, vegetables, B complex, gluten, sugar, iron, cold, heat, dried beans, spices, fats, grains, food additives.

ACUTAP/MASSAGE POINTS: St37(p.87), St25(p.38), CV6(p.39), NAET Ut(p.40), NAET UB(p.41), NAET LI(p.42), Kid3(p.98), Sp4(p.101).

55. CHEMICAL SENSITIVITY

COMMONLY SEEN ALLERGENS: Allergy to any food, drink, or chemical exposure you had couple of days before the symptoms started. Basic ten, proteins, calcium, vitamin C, citrus fruits, B complex, sugar, iron, hormones, trace minerals, carbonated drinks, ice cream, cold meats, chocolate, coffee, tea, fats, spices, artificial sweeteners, turkey, pollens, weeds, flowers, wood, smoke, cigarette smoke, emotional factors, chemicals, cleaning agents, gloves, bacteria, pesticides, formaldehyde, pen, pencil, newspaper, rings, wrist watch, stomach acids, base, heat, cold, and fabrics.

ACUTAP/MASSAGE POINTS: Liv3(p.102), Kid9(p.93), Liv5(p.95).

56. CHEST CONGESTION(lung congestion).

COMMONLY SEEN ALLERGENS: Allergy to any food, drink, or chemical exposure you had couple of days before the symptoms started. Basic ten, proteins, calcium, vitamin C, citrus fruits, B complex, sugar, iron, hormones, trace minerals, carbonated drinks, ice cream, cold meats, chocolate, coffee, tea, fats, spices, artificial sweeteners, turkey, pollens, weeds, flowers, wood, smoke, cigarette smoke, emotional factors, chemicals, cleaning agents, gloves, bacteria, pesticides, formaldehyde.

ACUTAP/MASSAGE POINTS: Lu5(p.45), Lu7(p.50), St40(p.90), Sp9(p.81).

57. CHEST PAINS(emotional, death, loss of job, relationship, etc.).

COMMONLY SEEN ALLERGENS: Loss of job, loss of relationship, loss of a loved one.

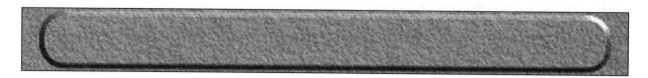

ACUTAP/MASSAGE POINTS: Pc6(p.46), Ht7(p.49), CV12(p.31), CV14(p.28).

58. CONSTIPATION

COMMONLY SEEN ALLERGENS: Basic ten, hormones, trace minerals, carbonated drinks, coffee, spices, artificial sweeteners, wood, smoke, cigarette smoke, emotional factors, chemicals, cleaning agents, gloves, bacteria, pesticides, formaldehyde.

ACUTAP/MASSAGE POINTS: St25(p.38), St36(p.83), St37(p.87), UB57(p.80), NAET LI(p.42).

59. COLD LIMBS

COMMONLY SEEN ALLERGENS: Basic ten, calcium, vitamin C, salt, B complex, sugar, iron, hormones, trace minerals, carbonated drinks, ice cream, cold meats, chocolate, coffee, tea, fats, spices, artificial sweeteners.

ACUTAP/MASSAGE POINTS: Sp6(p.96), St45(p.108), Kid3(p.98), Kid7(p.84), St36(p.83).

60. CHOKING WHILE YOU TALK TO STRANGERS (shyness)

COMMONLY SEEN ALLERGENS: Adrenal glands, kidney, B complex, sugar, trace minerals, food additives, food coloring.

ACUTAP/MASSAGE POINTS: E-Sweat(p.21), Ht5(p.48), SI4(p.52), Pc6(p.46).

61. CHRONIC FATIGUE SYNDROME

COMMONLY SEEN ALLERGENS: Basic ten, proteins, calcium, vitamin C, citrus fruits, B complex, sugar, iron, hormones, trace minerals, carbonated drinks, ice cream, cold meats, chocolate, coffee, tea, fats, spices, artificial sweeteners, turkey, pollens, weeds, flowers, wood, smoke, cigarette smoke, emotional factors, chemicals, cleaning agents, gloves, bacteria, pesticides, formaldehyde, pen, pencil, newspaper, rings, wrist watch, stomach acids, base, heat, cold, and fabrics.

ACUTAP/MASSAGE POINTS: Thymus(p.24), CV6(p.39), UB43(p.66), Sp10(p.75), Kid3(p.98), Kid7(p.94), LI11(p.44), Liv3(p.102), St36(p.83), Kid10(p.77), Liv5(p.95).

62. COMA/SEMI-CONSCIOUSNESS

COMMONLY SEEN ALLERGENS: Allergy to any food, drink, or chemical exposure you had before the symptoms started. Basic ten, hormones, trace minerals, carbonated drinks, coffee, spices, artificial sweeteners, wood, smoke, cigarette smoke, emotional factors, chemicals, cleaning agents, gloves, bacteria, pesticides, formaldehyde.

ACUTAP/MASSAGE POINTS: GV26(p.15), GV20(p.1), GB12(p.61), GB 20(p.63), LI1(p.56), Kid1(p.111), Pc9(p.58), Ht9(p.59).

63. COLITIS/IRRITABLE BOWELS

COMMONLY SEEN ALLERGENS: Basic ten, milk products, vitamin C, uncooked vegetables,

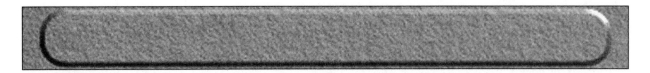

fruits, B complex, wheat, gluten, sugar, iron, cold, heat, dried beans, spices, salt, fats, turkey, grains, food additives, beds, sheets, detergents, fabrics, chemicals, pollens, weeds, flowers, and emotional blockages.

ACUTAP/MASSAGE POINTS: Sp6(p.96), St36(p.83), St25(p.38), GV4(p.72), CV12(p.31), Cv4(p.40), St37(p.87), Sp4(p.101), LI2(p.57).

64. COLD SORES

COMMONLY SEEN ALLERGENS: Basic ten, salt, citrus fruits, trace minerals, carbonated drinks, ice cream, cold meats, chocolate, coffee, tea, fats, spices, artificial sweeteners.

ACUTAP/MASSAGE POINTS: Sp10(p.75), CV12(p.31), St38(p.88), LI11(p.44), LI2(p.57).

65. COMMON COLD

COMMONLY SEEN ALLERGENS: Allergy to any food, drink, or chemical exposure you had before the symptoms started.

ACUTAP/MASSAGE POINTS: St8(p.3), GB20(p.63), GV14(p.4), LI20(p.14), GV24(p.2), GV20(p.1), St37(p.87), GB41(p.104).

66. CONVULSIONS

COMMONLY SEEN ALLERGENS: Allergy to any food, drink, or chemical exposure you had before the symptoms started.

ACUTAP/MASSAGE POINTS: GV26(p.15), Sp1(p.106), Liv8(p.78), Liv5(p.95), GV20(p.1), GB34(p.85), GB39(p.92).

67. COUGH

COMMONLY SEEN ALLERGENS: Basic ten, hormones, trace minerals, milk, carbonated drinks, coffee, spices, artificial sweeteners, wood, smoke, cigarette smoke, emotional factors, chemicals, cleaning agents, gloves, bacteria, pesticides, formaldehyde.

ACUTAP/MASSAGE POINTS: Lu1(p.25), St16(p.26), Lu7(p.50), Dingchuan(p.65), GV14(p.64), GV11(p.69), Lu11(p.55), St40(p.90), UB43(p.66).

68. CRAMPS IN THE LEGS (Charley horse)

COMMONLY SEEN ALLERGENS: Basic ten, cold drinks and foods, heat (humidity), dried beans, spices, fats, turkey, food additives (sulfites, whiten-all), kapok (pillow fills), mattress, pesticides, fabrics, detergents, fabric softeners, chemicals, vinyl, wood, metals, flowers, and emotional blockages.

ACUTAP/MASSAGE POINTS: UB39(p.76), UB57(p.80), St38(p.88), Sp9(p.81), GB39(p.92), Liv5(p.95).

69. CRAMPS IN THE LOWER ABDOMEN

COMMONLY SEEN ALLERGENS: Basic ten, hormones, carbonated drinks, coffee, spices,

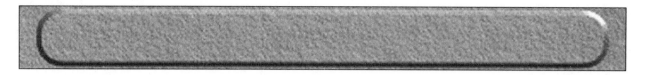

artificial sweeteners, wood, emotional factors, chemicals, bacteria, pesticides, formaldehyde.

ACUTAP/MASSAGE POINTS: St37(p.87), NAET Ut(p.40), LI2(p.57), LI4(p.53).

70. CROHN'S DISEASE/IRRITABLE BOWELS

COMMONLY SEEN ALLERGENS: Basic ten, whole grain, uncooked vegetable, uncooked fruit, carbonated drinks, coffee, spices, artificial sweeteners, wood, smoke, cigarette smoke, emotional factors, chemicals, cleaning agents, gloves, bacteria, pesticides, formaldehyde.

ACUTAP/MASSAGE POINTS: Sp4(p.101), St37(p.87), St25(p.38), CV4(p.40), St39(p.89).

71. CRYING SPELLS

COMMONLY SEEN ALLERGENS: Basic ten, proteins, milk products, wheat products, sugar products, tomato, spices, food additives, chemicals, alcohols, chemicals like chlorine, formaldehyde, fabric softeners, dry cereals, metals, vinyl, leather, ear phones, ear plugs, ear wax.

ACUTAP/MASSAGE POINTS: NAET Liv(p.34), CV17(p.27), Pc6(p.46), Ht7(p.49), Ht5(p.48), CV14(p.28).

72. DEAFNESS AND RINGING IN THE EAR

COMMONLY SEEN ALLERGENS: Basic ten, proteins, milk products, wheat products, sugar products, tomato, spices, food additives, chemicals, alcohols, formaldehyde, fabric softeners, dry cereals, metals, vinyl, leather, ear phones, ear plugs, ear wax.

ACUTAP/MASSAGE POINTS: Lu9(p.51), UB23(p.73), SI3(p.54), TH5(p.47), Kid3(p.98), St7(p.11), SI19(p.9), GB2(p.10).

73. DEPRESSION

COMMONLY SEEN ALLERGENS: Basic ten, proteins, milk products, vitamin C products, wheat products, sugar products, trace minerals, tomato, spices, food additives, city water, fluoride, alcohol, chemicals like chlorine, formaldehyde, different fabrics, cotton, polyester, fabric softeners, metals, vinyl, leather.

ACUTAP/MASSAGE POINTS: Sp6(p.96), St41(p.97), LI11(p.44), CV12(p.31), Pc6(p.46), E-shenmen(p.22), Ht7(p.49).

74. DIARRHEA

COMMONLY SEEN ALLERGENS: Basic ten, water, parasites, proteins, milk products, wheat products, sugar products, tomato, spices, food additives, alcohols, chemicals like chlorine, formaldehyde, fabric softeners, dry cereals, metals, vinyl, leather.

ACUTAP/MASSAGE POINTS: St25(p.38), CV8(p.36), GV4(p.72). Kid16(p.37), CV12(p.31), CV6(p.39), UB20(p.71), LI11(p.44), Sp8(p.82), St37(p.87), St36(p.83), Liv3(p.102), UB40(p.79), Sp1(p.106).

75. DIFFICULTY IN BREATHING

COMMONLY SEEN ALLERGENS: Water, parasites, Basic ten, proteins, milk products, wheat products, sugar products, tomato, spices, food additives, chemicals, alcohols, chemicals like chlorine, formaldehyde, fabric softeners, dry cereals, metals, vinyl, leather.

ACUTAP/MASSAGE POINTS: GV26(p.15), GB12(p.61), Lu1(p.25), E-Asthma(p.20), St16(26), CV6(39), Kid27(p.29), Lu11(55), GV14(p.64), Lu5(p.45), Lu7(p.50), UB43(p.66), St40(p.90), Kid3(p.98), CV17(p.27), Dingchuan(p.65).

76. DIFFICULTY IN SWALLOWING

COMMONLY SEEN ALLERGENS: Water, Basic ten, proteins, milk products, wheat products, sugar products, tomato, spices, food additives, alcohols, chemicals like chlorine, formaldehyde, fabric softeners, dry cereals, metals, vinyl, leather.

ACUTAP/MASSAGE POINTS: CV14(p.28), CV17(p.27), SI3(p.54), GV14(p.64), CV12(p.31), NAET Liv(p.34), Kid9(p.93).

77. DIFFICULTY IN URINATING

COMMONLY SEEN ALLERGENS: Water, Basic ten, proteins, milk products, wheat products, sugar products, tomato, spices, food additives, chemicals, alcohols, chemicals like chlorine, formaldehyde, fabric softeners, dry cereals, metals, vinyl, leather.

ACUTAP/MASSAGE POINTS: NAET UB(p.41), Liv8(p.78), UB39(p.76), Sp9(p.81), Sp8(p.82), Liv5(p.95), Liv1(p.107).

78. DISCOLORATION OF THE SCLERA

COMMONLY SEEN ALLERGENS: Spices, fish, sugar, dust, water, fumes, exhaust, grasses, weeds, pollens, eyeglasses, contact lenses.

ACUTAP/MASSAGE POINTS: SI18(p.9), GB14(p.4), St2(p.13), yintang(p.5), Taiyang(p.7).

79. DIVERTICULITIS

COMMONLY SEEN ALLERGENS: Basic ten, uncooked grain, uncooked vegetable, uncooked fruit, proteins, milk products, wheat products, sugar products, tomato, spices, food additives, parasites, water chemicals, alcohol, formaldehyde, fabric softeners, dry cereals.

ACUTAP/MASSAGE POINTS: Sp4(p.101), St37(p.87), GV20(p.1), St25(p.38), NAET LI(p.42).

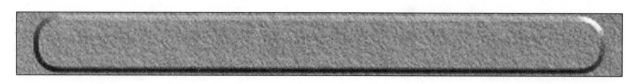

80. DIZZINESS

COMMONLY SEEN ALLERGENS: Basic ten, proteins, calcium, vitamin C, citrus fruits, B complex, sugar, iron, hormones, trace minerals, carbonated drinks, ice cream, cold meats, chocolate, coffee, tea, fats, spices, artificial sweeteners, turkey, pollens, weeds, flowers, wood, smoke, cigarette smoke, emotional factors, chemicals, cleaning agents, gloves, bacteria, pesticides, formaldehyde, pen, pencil, newspaper, rings, wrist watch, stomach acids, base, heat, cold, and fabrics.

ACUTAP/MASSAGE POINTS: Thymus(p.24), CV6(p.39), UB43(p.66), Sp10(p.75), Kid3(p.98), Kid7(p.94), LI11(p.44), Liv3(p.102), St 36(p.83), KId10(p.77), Liv5(p.95).

81. NIGHTMARES

COMMONLY SEEN ALLERGENS: Basic ten, proteins, milk products, wheat products, sugar products, tomato, spices, food additives, parasites, water chemicals, alcohol, formaldehyde, fabric softeners, dry cereals.

ACUTAP/MASSAGE POINTS: Sp1(p.106), St37(p.87), GB44(p.109), St45(p.108).

82. DRYNESS OF THE MOUTH

COMMONLY SEEN ALLERGENS: Basic ten, beverages like tea, coffee, chocolate, fruits (like citrus), vegetables (artichoke, asparagus, carrot), salt, sugar products, breads, gums, raisins, food additives.

ACUTAP/MASSAGE POINTS: CV24(p.17), GV26(p.15), Sp6(p.96), Sp10(p.75), H7(p.49), CV12(p.31), CV6(p.39), CV17(p.27).

83. DRYNESS OF THE TONGUE

COMMONLY SEEN ALLERGENS: Milk products, wheat products, sugar products, tomato, spices, food additives, water chemicals, alcohol, dentures, tooth paste, tooth brush, mouth wash.

ACUTAP/MASSAGE POINTS: Kid1(p.111), sympathetic(p.21), CV24(p.17), GV20(p.1), GV26(p.15), LI20(p.14).

84. DYSENTERY

COMMONLY SEEN ALLERGENS: Basic ten, proteins, milk products, wheat products, sugar products, tomato, spices, food additives, parasites, water chemicals, alcohol, formaldehyde, fabric softeners, dry cereals.

ACUTAP/MASSAGE POINTS: St25(p.38), CV12(p.31), UB20(p.71), LI11(p.44), St37(p.87), Sp8(p.82), Sp1(p.106).

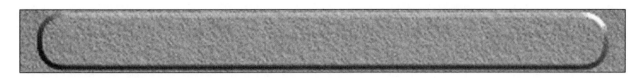

85. DYSMENORRHEA

COMMONLY SEEN ALLERGENS: Basic ten, proteins, milk products, wheat products, sugar products, tomato, spices, chocolate, caffeine, hormones, salt.

ACUTAP/MASSAGE POINTS: NAET Ut(p.40), Sp6(p.96), Pc6(p.46), LI4(p.53), Liv3(p.102).

86. EARACHE

COMMONLY SEEN ALLERGENS: Allergy to any food, drink, chemical exposure, you had within 24-48 hours, milk products, wheat products, sugar products, tomato, spices, chocolate, caffeine, soft drinks, chlorine.

ACUTAP/MASSAGE POINTS: St7(p.11), SI19(p.8), TH5(p.47), LI 11(p.44), Kid9(p.93).

87. EAR INFECTION

COMMONLY SEEN ALLERGENS: Allergy to any food, drink, chemical exposure, you had within 24-48 hours, milk products, wheat products, sugar products, tomato, spices, chocolate, caffeine, soft drinks, chlorine.

ACUTAP/MASSAGE POINTS: St7(p.11), SI19(p.8), TH5(p.47), LI 11(p.44), Kid9(p.93).

88. EATING DISORDERS

COMMONLY SEEN ALLERGENS: Basic ten, proteins, milk products, vitamin C products, wheat products, sugar products, trace minerals, zinc, vitamin B12, phenolics, stomach acids, digestive enzymes, fish and shell fish, alcohol, artificial sweeteners, water, food colors as in lipsticks, emotional upsets, emotional blockages.

ACUTAP/MASSAGE POINTS: CV12(p.31), St36(p.83), Sp6(p.96), LI4(p.53), Liv3(p.102), LI11(p.44), Pc6(p.46), Ear-shenmen(p.22).

89. ECZEMA

COMMONLY SEEN ALLERGENS: Basic ten, proteins, milk products, vitamin C products, wheat products, sugar products, fish and shell fish, nuts, prescription drugs, vitamin supplements, herbs, trace minerals, fruits, corn, starches, chromium, parasites, city water, vegetable and animal fats, chewing gums, candy, chocolate, food additives, cosmetics, body lotions, detergents, fabric softeners, fabrics, carpets, pets, lactic acid, sweat, heat, humidity.

ACUTAP/MASSAGE POINTS: Sp10(p.75), Liv8(p.78), UB40(p.79), GB2(p.10), LI11(p.44), Pc6(p.46).

90. EDEMA

COMMONLY SEEN ALLERGENS: Basic ten, proteins, milk products, vitamin C, vegetables like zucchini, squash, fruits like citrus, berries, soft drinks, table salt, nuts, fats, fish, turkey, food additives, food colors, fabrics, chemicals, water chemicals.

ACUTAP/MASSAGE POINTS: CV6(p.39), Sp9(p.81), St40(p.90), St 25(p.38), UB57(p.80), Sp8(p.82).

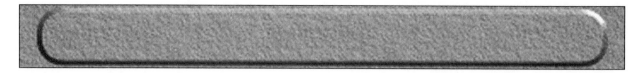

91. ELECTRIC AND ELECTRO-MAGNETIC ENERGY IMBALANCES

COMMONLY SEEN ALLERGENS: Basic ten, vitamin D, pineal gland, magnet, salt, electric outlets, electric bulbs, lamps, cords, microwave, radio, T.V., electric blankets, hair dryer, cosmetic devices, electric shaver, tooth brush, washer, dryer, any other electric equipment.

ACUTAP/MASSAGE POINTS: Yintang(p.5), Pc6(p.46), LI11(p.44), GB14(p.14), GV20(p.1), GV26(p.15), GV11(p.69).

92. ENVIRONMENTAL TOXICITY/ SICK BUILDING SYNDROME

COMMONLY SEEN ALLERGENS: Basic ten, Chemicals, odors, fumes, perfumes, new clothes, formaldehyde, leather, water chemicals, pesticides, pollens, weeds, flowers, dust, paints, building materials, mold, animals, insects like cockroaches, fleas, etc.

ACUTAP/MASSAGE POINTS: Liv3(p.102), LU1(p.25), LI20(p.14), UB43(p.66), GB20(p.63), GV26(p.15), GV20(p.1), Liv5(p.95).

93. EYE INFLAMMATION (Red eye).

COMMONLY SEEN ALLERGENS: Basic ten, fish, food additives, smoke, cosmetics, fumes, pollens, incense.

ACUTAP/MASSAGE POINTS: St2(p.13), UB2(p.12), GB37(p.91).

94. EYE INFECTIONS

COMMONLY SEEN ALLERGENS: Basic ten, fish, food additives, wood smoke, city water, chlorine, soft drinks, cosmetics, fumes of different kind, wind, pollens, incense.

ACUTAP/MASSAGE POINTS: Taiyang(p.7), LI11(p.44), UB40(p.79), E-eye(p.18), GB37(p.91), St2(p.13), GB44(p.109), UB2(p.12), UB67(p.110).

95. EYE PAIN

COMMONLY SEEN ALLERGENS: Basic ten, fish, food additives, smoke, chemicals, soft drinks, cosmetics, food coloring, pillow, fumes, news- paper inks, old books, T.V.

ACUTAP/MASSAGE POINTS: Taiyang(p.7), E-Eye(p.18), St2(p.13), UB2(p.12), SI18(p.9), GB2(p.10).

96. EYE STRESS

COMMONLY SEEN ALLERGENS: Basic ten, vitamin A, iron, chromium, sugar, insulin, eye glasses, books and lack of vitamin A.

ACUTAP/MASSAGE POINTS: E-eye(p.18), St2(p.13), UB2(p.12), GB39(p.92), GB37(p.91), GB44(p.109).

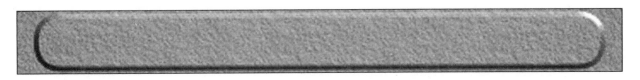

97. EPILEPSY

COMMONLY SEEN ALLERGENS: Basic ten, proteins, milk products, vitamin C products, wheat products, sugar products, trace minerals, fish and shell fish, nuts, prescription drugs, vitamin supplements, corn, starches, chromium, parasites, vegetable oils, animal fats, chewing gums, candy, chocolate, food additives, cosmetics, body lotions, detergents, fabric softeners, fabrics, carpets, pets, lactic acid, pesticides.

ACUTAP/MASSAGE POINTS: GV20(p.1), GV26(p.15), NAET GB(p.35), NAET Liv(p.34), CV14(p.28), GV14(p.64), SI3(p.54), St40(p.90), Liv 3(p.102), Kid6(p.100), UB60(p.99), Liv1(p.107), UB15(p.70), Sp4(p.101).

98. EBV (Epstein-barr virus disease)

COMMONLY SEEN ALLERGENS: Basic ten, tap water, proteins, milk products, vitamin C products, wheat products, sugar products, trace minerals, fish and shell fish, corn, starches, parasites, animal fats, food additives, detergents, fabric softeners, fabrics, carpets, pets, pesticides.

ACUTAP/MASSAGE POINTS: Thymus(p.24), Sp10(p.75), LI11(p.44), St36(p.83), Liv5(p.95), NAET Sp(p.32), UB40(p.79).

99. EXCESSIVE PERSPIRATION/ ABNORMAL PERSPIRATION

COMMONLY SEEN ALLERGENS: Basic ten, adrenal gland, thyroid gland, prostaglandin, phenolics, tap water, proteins, milk products, vitamin C products, wheat products, sugar products, trace minerals, fish and shell fish, corn, starches, parasites, animal fats, food additives, hormones, heat, detergents, fabric softeners, fabrics, carpets, pets, pesticides.

ACUTAP/MASSAGE POINTS: E-Sweat(p.21), LI11(p.44), GV14(p.64), Liv 8(p.78), Kid7(p.94), St8(p.3).

100. FAINTING

COMMONLY SEEN ALLERGENS: Basic ten, water, food, iron, soy products, sugar, fumes, formaldehyde, salt, alcohol, emotions.

ACUTAP/MASSAGE POINTS: GV26(p.15), LI1(p.56), P9(p.58), Ht9(p.59), Kid1(p.111), GB12(p.61).

101. FEVER

COMMONLY SEEN ALLERGENS: Basic ten, tap water, proteins, milk products, vitamin C products, wheat products, sugar products, trace minerals, fish and shell fish, corn, starches, parasites, animal fats, food additives, hormones, heat, detergents, fabric softeners, fabrics, carpets, pets, pesticides.

ACUTAP/MASSAGE POINTS: Lu9(p.51), LI4(p.53), SI3(p.54), Pc9(p.58), UB39(p.76), GB20(p.63), GV14(p.64), LI11(p.44), GB44(p.109), St44(p.104), St45(p.108), UB60(p.99), Kid1(p.111).

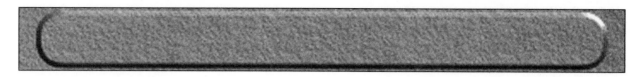

102. FIBROMYALGIA

COMMONLY SEEN ALLERGENS: Basic ten, proteins, calcium, magnesium, phosphorus, vitamin D, B complex vitamins, sugar, yeast, candida, parasites, vitamin F, alcohol, starches, spices, fabrics, fabric softener, chemicals, formaldehyde.

ACUTAP/MASSAGE POINTS: Sp21(p.30), Sp6(p.96), Sp10(p.75), St36(p.83), LI4(p.53), LI11(p.44), Liv3(p.102), CV6(p.39), Pc6(p.46), CV17(p.27).

103. FOOD POISONING

COMMONLY SEEN ALLERGENS: Get a sample of the exact food, if that is not possible collect a small sample of the person's vomit, take this sample to your nearest NAET doctor. In the meanwhile, use these points to treat yourself.

ACUTAP/MASSAGE POINTS: CV12(p.31), Pc6(p.46), St36(p.83), Liv3(p.102), CV6(p.39), Sp4(p.101), NAET SI(p.36), CV17(p.27), St25(p.38), St44(p.103), Sp9(p.81), Kid3(p.98), GV4(p.72), NAET Sp(p.32), St37(p.87).

104. GENERAL BODY ACHE

COMMONLY SEEN ALLERGENS: Basic ten, proteins, calcium, vitamin D, fruits, B complex vitamins, sugar, magnesium, phosphorus, sodium, potassium, grains, yeast, candida, parasites, vitamin F, alcohol, starches, spices, fabrics, fabric softener, chemicals, formaldehyde.

ACUTAP/MASSAGE POINTS: Sp21(p.30), Liv5(p.95), Pc6(p.46), St36(p.83), Sp6(p.96), LI11(p.44), Liv1(p.107).

105. GALL BLADDER PAIN

COMMONLY SEEN ALLERGENS: Basic ten, proteins, calcium, vitamin D, fruits, B complex vitamins, sugar, fats, deep fried food. water, grains, yeast, candida, parasites, vitamin F.

ACUTAP/MASSAGE POINTS: Dannang (p.86), NAET GB(p.35)), GB34(p.85), Pc6(p.46), Ht7(p.49), St25(p.38).

106. HEAT STROKE

COMMONLY SEEN ALLERGENS: Exposure to extreme heat, lack of liquids.

ACUTAP/MASSAGE POINTS: GV26(p.15), Pc9(p.58), GV14(p.64).

107. HEAT SENSATION IN THE SOLE

COMMONLY SEEN ALLERGENS: Anything you drank or ate within 24 hours, Basic ten, socks, shoes.

ACUTAP/MASSAGE POINTS: UB67(p.110), Kid1(p.111), TH5(p.47).

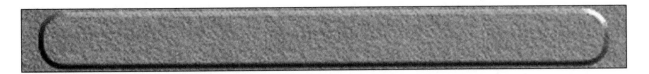

108. HEART IRREGULARITIES

COMMONLY SEEN ALLERGENS: Basic ten, calcium, vitamin D, salt, food additives, food coloring, sulfites, caffeine, alcohols, fruits, tomato, whiten-all, B.complex vitamins, sugar, wheat, corn, yeast, vegetable fats, animal fats, spices, chocolate, artificial sweeteners, nuts, starches, fabrics, chemicals.

ACUTAP/MASSAGE POINTS: GV20(p.1), GV11(p.69), GV26(p.15), Ht7(p.49), Pc6(p.46), Pc9(p.58), Dingchuan(p.65),

109. HYPOGLYCEMIA

COMMONLY SEEN ALLERGENS: Basic ten, proteins, calcium, vitamin D, fruits, B complex vitamins, sugar, magnesium, phosphorus, sodium, potassium, grains, yeast, candida, corn, insulin, pancreas, parasites, vitamin F, alcohol, starches, spices, fabrics, fabric softener, chemicals, formaldehyde.

ACUTAP/MASSAGE POINTS: NAET Pan(p.33), NAET Sp(p.32), CV12(p.31), Sp9(p.81), LI4(p.53), UB39(p.76), LI11(p.44), St36(p.83), Liv3 (p.102), E-Sweat(p.21), Yintang(p.5), Sp1(p.106), Pc6(p.46).

110. HEADACHES (In general)

COMMONLY SEEN ALLERGENS: Basic ten, proteins, calcium, vitamin D, fruits, B complex vitamins, sugar, wheat, corn, yeast, vegetable fats, animal fats, spices, chocolate, artificial sweeteners, food additives, food coloring, caffeine, alcohols, starches, fabrics, chemicals.

ACUTAP/MASSAGE POINTS: St8(p.3), GV24(p.2), GV20(p.1), GV26(p.15), GB21(p.23), GB20(p.63), LI20(p.14), Yintang(p.5).

111. HEADACHE, MIGRAINES (One sided headaches- Gall bladder headache).

COMMONLY SEEN ALLERGENS: Basic ten, proteins, milk products, vitamin C products, B complex vitamins, sugar, calcium, sodium, phosphorus, magnesium, hormones, iron, salt, stomach acid, base, vitamin D, digestive enzymes, potassium, wheat, corn, yeast, yogurt, whey, superheated oils, vegetable fats, animal fats, alcohols, cold.

ACUTAP/MASSAGE POINTS: St8(p.3), GB1(p.6), GB34(p.85), GB41(p.104), UB2(p.12), GB19(p.61), GB20(p.63), GV24(p.2).

112. HEADACHE, MIGRAINES (Top of the head - Liver headache).

COMMONLY SEEN ALLERGENS: Basic ten, Proteins, milk products, vitamin C products, B complex vitamins, sugar, calcium, food additives, chemicals, pesticides, formaldehyde, hormones, boron, iron, salt, stomach acid, base, vitamin D, digestive enzymes, potassium, wheat, corn, yeast, yogurt, whey, heated vegetable fats and animal fats, alcohols, cold.

ACUTAP/MASSAGE POINTS: GV20(p.1), St8(p.3), GB1(p.6), GB34(p.85), GB41(p.104), UB2(p.12), GB19(p.61), GB20(p.63).

113. HEADACHE, MIGRAINES (Front of the head, or forehead and eyes - stomach headache).

COMMONLY SEEN ALLERGENS: Basic ten, Proteins, milk products, vitamin C products, B complex vitamins, sugar, stomach acids, spices, food colors, salt, iodine, heat, cold, vitamin D, digestive enzymes, wheat, corn, yeast, yogurt, whey, heated vegetable fats and animal fats, alcohols, smoke, perfumes, nicotine, recreational drugs.

ACUTAP/MASSAGE POINTS: St8(p.3), UB2(p.12), LI20(p.14), Yintang(p.5), GV24(p.2), GB14(p.4), St41(p.97), St36(p.83), St37(p.87), LI4(p.53), LI11(p.44), CV12(p.31).

114. HEADACHE, MIGRAINES (Back of the head, Bladder headache).

COMMONLY SEEN ALLERGENS: Basic ten, proteins, milk products, vitamin C products, B complex vitamins, sugar, tomato, corn, feather pillow, name tags on the clothes, stomach acids, spices, food colors, salt, iodine, heat, cold, vitamin D, digestive enzymes, wheat, corn, yeast, yogurt, whey, heated vegetable fats and animal fats, alcohols, smoke, perfumes, nicotine, cocaine, recreational drugs.

ACUTAP/MASSAGE POINTS: UB2(p.12), LI20(p.14), GB19(p.61), GB20(p.63), GV14(p.64), GV20(p.1), UB40(p.79), UB60(p.99), Kid3(p.98), LI4(p.53), LI11(p.44).

115. HEARTBURN

COMMONLY SEEN ALLERGENS: Basic ten, proteins, calcium, vitamin D, fruits, B complex vitamins, sugar, wheat, corn, yeast, vegetable fats, animal fats, spices, chocolate, artificial sweeteners, nuts, food additives, food coloring, caffeine, alcohols, starches, fabrics, chemicals.

ACUTAP/MASSAGE POINTS: CV12(p.31), Pc6(p.46), St36(p.83), St39(p.89), Liv5(p.95).

116. HIGH BLOOD PRESSURE

COMMONLY SEEN ALLERGENS: Basic ten, proteins, calcium, vitamin D, fruits, B complex vitamins, sugar, salt, potassium, wheat, corn, yeast, vegetable fats, animal fats, spices, chocolate, artificial sweeteners, nuts, food additives, food coloring, caffeine, alcohols, starches, fabrics, chemicals.

ACUTAP/MASSAGE POINTS: kid9(p.93), GV20(p.1), Liv3(p.102), LI 11(p.44), LI4(p.53), St36(p.83), Liv5(p.95), Anmian(p.62), GB20(p.63).

117. HIVES

COMMONLY SEEN ALLERGENS: Basic ten, Tomato, fish, shellfish, fruits, milk products, corn, salt, sugar, food additives, food colors, yeast, chocolate, fabrics, chemicals, cleansing chemicals, weeds, grasses, poison ivy, peaches, cashew nuts, onions, melons, peppers, spices.

ACUTAP/MASSAGE POINTS: UB40(p.79), LI11(p.44), Sp10(p.75), LI4(p.53), St25(p.38).

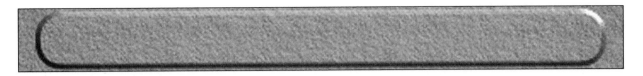

118. INDIGESTION

COMMONLY SEEN ALLERGENS: Basic ten, proteins, milk products, vitamin D, fruits, B complex vitamins, sugar, salt, stomach acid, base, digestive enzymes, potassium, wheat, corn, yeast, vegetable fats, animal fats, spices, chocolate, artificial sweeteners, nuts, food additives, food coloring, caffeine, alcohols, starches, fabrics, chemicals.

ACUTAP/MASSAGE POINTS: CV12(p.31), St25(p.38), St44(p.103), CV14(p.28), St36(p.83).

119. INSOMNIA

COMMONLY SEEN ALLERGENS: Basic ten, Proteins, milk products, vitamin D, fruits, B complex vitamins, sugar, salt, stomach acid, base, digestive enzymes, potassium, wheat, corn, yeast, vegetable fats, animal fats, spices, chocolate, artificial sweeteners, nuts, food additives, food coloring, caffeine, alcohols, starches, fabrics, chemicals.

ACUTAP/MASSAGE POINTS: GV20(p.1), Ht7(p.49), Kid6(p.100), Liv8(p.78), Sp9(p.81), Kid3(p.98), NAET Liv(p.34), Anmian(p.62), Sp4(p.101), Ht5(p.48).

120. LARYNGITIS

COMMONLY SEEN ALLERGENS: Anything you drank or ate within 24-48 hours, Basic ten, Fruits, lemon, fish, shellfish, fats, fabrics like wool, polyester, chemicals, emotions.

ACUTAP/MASSAGE POINTS: Kid1(p.111), Thymus(p.24), CV17(p.27), LU11(p.55).

121. LEAKY GUT SYNDROME

COMMONLY SEEN ALLERGENS: Basic ten, whole grain, uncooked vegetable, uncooked fruit, proteins, carbonated drinks, coffee, spices, smoke, emotional factors, bacteria, pesticide, parasites.

ACUTAP/MASSAGE POINTS: Sp4(p.101), St37(p.87), St25(p.38), CV4(p.40), Sp6(p.96), Cv12(p.31), St38(p.88).

122. LOW ENERGY

COMMONLY SEEN ALLERGENS: Anything you drank or ate within 24-48 hours, Basic ten, Proteins, milk products, vitamin C products, B complex vitamins, sugar, stomach acids, spices, food colors, salt, iodine, heat, cold, vitamin D, digestive enzymes, wheat, corn, yeast, yogurt, whey, heated vegetable fats and animal fats, alcohols, smoke, perfumes, nicotine, recreational drugs.

ACUTAP/MASSAGE POINTS: GV20(p.1), GV26(p.15), UB23(p.71), UB43(p.66), Kid7(p.94), Liv5(p.95), Liv3(p.102), St36(p.83), CV17(p.27), CV6(p.39).

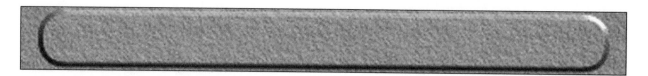

123. MENSTRUATION, DIFFICULT(Pre-menstrual disorders/PMS)

COMMONLY SEEN ALLERGENS: Basic ten, Iron, calcium, B complex, foods and drinks ingested during the last 48 hours, salt, emotional blockages.

ACUTAP/MASSAGE POINTS: CV4(P.40), LI4(p.53), Sp10(p.75), Sp8(p.82), Liv3(p.102), St36(p.83), Sp6(p.96).

124. NAUSEA/MORNING SICKNESS

COMMONLY SEEN ALLERGENS: Basic ten, Iron, calcium, B complex, foods and drinks ingested during the last 48 hours, emotions, nausea as in chemotherapy, radiation treatment, morning sickness etc.

ACUTAP/MASSAGE POINTS: CV12(p.31), PC6(p.46).

125. OVERACTIVE MIND (Cannot stop thinking)

COMMONLY SEEN ALLERGENS: Anything you drank or ate within 24-48 hours, Basic ten, Proteins, milk products, vitamin C products, B complex vitamins, sugar, stomach acids, spices, food colors, salt, iodine, heat, cold, vitamin D, digestive enzymes, wheat, corn, yeast, yogurt, whey, heated vegetable fats and animal fats, alcohols, smoke, perfumes, nicotine, recreational drugs.

ACUTAP/MASSAGE POINTS: Yintang(p.5), Pc6(p.46), Ht5(p.48), GV20(p.1).

126. RESTLESS LEG SYNDROME

COMMONLY SEEN ALLERGENS: Chemicals in food or drink, fabrics, chemicals in the fabrics, Basic ten, cotton, polyester, detergents, fabric softeners, perfumes.

ACUTAP/MASSAGE POINTS: St38(p.88), GV20(p.1), GV26(p.15), UB23(p.71), Liv5(p.95), Liv3(p.102), St36(p.83), CV17(p.27), CV6(p.39).

127. SCIATIC NEURALGIA

COMMONLY SEEN ALLERGENS: Anything you drank or ate within 24-48 hours, Basic ten, cold, heat, dried beans, spices, fats, turkey, potato, milk products, tomato, bell pepper, gelatin, beds, sheets, detergents, fabrics, elastics, chemicals, furniture, desk, wood, and emotional blockages.

ACUTAP/MASSAGE POINTS: UB 40(p.79), GV26(P.15), LI2(p.57), GV4(p.72), GV3(p.74), PC6(p.46).

128. SHORTNESS OF BREATH

COMMONLY SEEN ALLERGENS: Any food or drink 0-24 hours before the attack, basic ten, milk products, fruits, vegetables, eggs or egg products, food additives, whiten-all, turkey, food colors, alcohols, corn, grain, nuts, tea, coffee, dried beans, proteins, cosmetics, talcum powder, baking powder, honey, sugar products, cinnamon, fumes, perfumes, gasoline, mold, grass, weeds, paper, ink, fabrics, chemicals, water chemicals, onions, peppers, egg plants, tomato, potato, cheese, ice cream.

ACUTAP/MASSAGE POINTS: Lu1(p.25), St16(p.26), CV6(p.39), Lu11(p.55), GV14(p.64), Lu5(p.45), Lu7(p.50), UB43(p.66), St40(p.90), Kid3(p.98), CV17(p.27), E-asthma(p.20), Dingchuan(p.65).

129. SORE THROAT

COMMONLY SEEN ALLERGENS: Any food or drink within 0-24 hours, milk, basic ten, milk products, lemonade, juices, vitamin C products, cold direct breeze, water chemicals from the water, pesticides, fabric softeners, detergent, chemical spray, perfumes, fried foods, heated oils, turkey, chocolate, cotton candy, cold drinks in hot weather, air-conditioning, natural gas heating, carpets, paints, fish, chewing gum, glue.

ACUTAP/MASSAGE POINTS: Lu11(p.55), LI4(p.53), St44(p.103), Kid3(p.98), Lu7(p.50). LI20(p.14), LI11(p.44), Liv3(p.102)

130. TOOTHACHE

COMMONLY SEEN ALLERGENS: Any food or drink within 0-24 hours, basic ten, milk products, sugar products, artificial sweeteners, spices, nuts, yeast, food additives, food colors, dental anaesthesia, tooth brush, tooth paste, gargles,

ACUTAP/MASSAGE POINTS: LI4(p.53), St44(p.103), St7(p.11), TH5(p.47), Kid3(p.98).

131. UNABLE TO CRY(Due to overwhelming emotions)

COMMONLY SEEN ALLERGENS: Winning lottery, sudden loss of a loved one, sudden loss of a large amount of money.

ACUTAP/MASSAGE POINTS: Ht7(p.49), NAETLiv(p.34), NAETGB(p.35), St16(p.26), CV17(p.27), Ht7(p.49), PC6(p.46), SI4(p.52).

132. NERVOUSNESS OF ALL KINDS(Pre-nuptial jitters, nervousness before job interview, taking an exam, your first date, first day at school, first day at your first job, etc).

ACUTAP/MASSAGE POINTS: E-sweat(p.21), E-shenmen(p.22), PC6(p.46), Ht7(p.49), CV12(p.31), CV17(p.27), SI4(p.52).

CHAPTER 4

GENERAL BALANCING POINTS

Massage these points (Rt 53, Rt 44, 15, Lt 44, Lt 53, Lt 102, Rt 102, Rt 53) for 1 minute clockwise twice a day. Please look up the positions of the points carefully. Treating these points will increase your overall energy.
Massage the points in the above order.

These are the additional points used for balancing the energy. After the above treatment you may use these points in any order: 27, 39, 49.

A point stimulator may be used in place of finger massage.

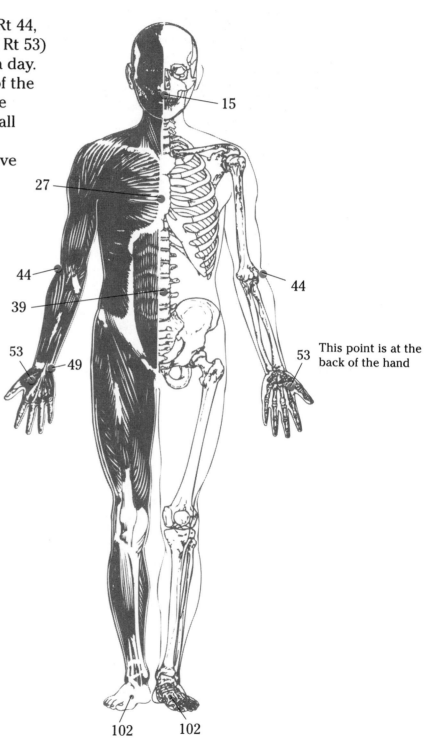

15

27

44

39

44

53

49

53   This point is at the back of the hand

102   102

CHAPTER 5

Acupressure
Therapeutic Points
without Illustrations

This chapter contains many frequently seen health disorders without illustrations. If you are suffering from one of these health disorders, you may stimulate the points that correspond with that disorder. Point locations are shown on pages 13 and 14. Follow the acupressure techniques you learned in chapter 1. If you are pregnant or if you have a pace maker, please do not use the point stimulator.

Abnormal salivation: 16, 17, 50, 51.
Connective tissue disorders: 1, 24, 84, 85, 92, 95.
Constant allergic reactions: 24, 52, 75, 77, 79.
Decreased white blood cell count: 24, 31, 51, 75, 95, 96.
Delayed menstrual cycles: 53, 75, 96.
Dental anaesthesia: 53, 104.
Deviation of the eye: 6, 7, 9, 12, 13, 91, 104.
Deviation of the mouth: 7, 8, 9, 11, 14, 15, 16, 17, 108.
Diabetes: 15, 33, 44, 75, 76, 83.
Drooling: 16, 17, 46, 71.
Drooping of the eyelids: 4, 7, 13, 14, 15.
Emphysema: 24, 25, 27, 28, 30, 31, 65, 66.
Enlargement of the breast in male: 78, 94, 98, 103.
Facial palsy: 3, 6, 7, 9, 11, 13, 14, 15, 16, 17, 46, 61.
Failing vision: 9, 10, 12, 13, 18, 79, 91, 92, 109 , 110.
Failing memory: 1, 2, 43, 38, 58, 59, 60, 63, 66, 77, 83, 96.
Falling eyebrow: 31, 77, 79, 87, 95.
Falling hair: 31, 77, 79, 87, 95, 102.
Far sightedness: 7, 9, 10, 12, 13, 18, 91, 92, 109.
Fat intolerance: 31, 35, 85,
Fear of darkness: 21, 46, 48, 52, 98.
Fear of strangers: 21, 46, 48, 52, 98.

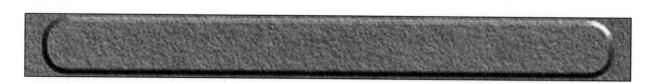

Fear in general: 46, 48, 98.
Fear in children: 46, 48, 98, 106.
Fever without sweating: 64.
Flatulence: 31, 36, 38, 42.
Food retention: 31, 44, 104.
Forgetfullness: 68.
Frequency of urination: 40, 41, 98, 100.
Frozen shoulder: 23, 25, 44, 45, 67, 68.
Gastric Ulcer: 31, 46, 83, 101.
Glaucoma: 4, 6, 12, 54.
Hair loss in men: 77, 78, 79.
Hair loss in women: 32, 77, 78, 95, 96.
Hairloss due to chemotherapy: 1, 77, 79, 95.
Hand tremor: 47, 85.
Hay-fever: 14, 25, 35.
Hiccup: 27, 93.
High creatinine in the blood: 93.
High cholesterol in the blood: 34, 44, 53, 102.
High sodium intake: 93.
High Triglycerides: 44, 75, 83, 95.
High blood urea nitrogen in the blood: 93.
Hoarse voice: 48, 108
Hodgkin's disease: 24, 51, 75
Hormone imbalance in female or male: 32, 96, 78.
Hot palms and soles: 65, 76.
Hot flashes: 31, 36, 47, 76, 96.
Hyperacidity: 5, 21, 62, 106.
Immature blood cell production: 24, 75.
Immune deficiency disorders: 24, 66, 75, 95, 96, 101.
Impotence: 36, 72, 73, 74, 77, 84, 96, 98, 100.
Improve memory: 5, 15, 46, 49, 98.
Improve psychic ability: 5, 100.
Improve yang energy in older people: 94.
Infertility in male: 78, 96.
Internal hemorrhage: 46, 49, 96, 100.
Irritability: 46, 49, 55, 70.
Itchy eyes: 44, 53, 91.
Itching of the body: 44, 53, 75, 78, 95.
Jet lag: 5, 21, 46.
Jock itch: 44, 46, 78, 95.
Kidney infection: 50, 75, 81, 96.
Kidney not able to filter enough urine: 78, 81, 95, 96.
Lactation deficiency: 26, 27.
Leukemia: 24, 32, 75.

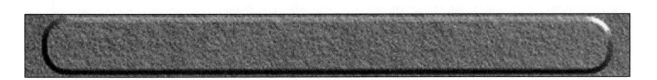

To live long: 83.
Liver flukes: 34, 35, 38, 42, 86.
Long term sickness: 1, 15, 24, 66, 71, 83, 94, 95, 102.
Loose stools with undigested food: 96.
Loss of consciousness: 15, 55, 56, 58, 59, 111.
Low platelets: 24, 32, 75.
Low red blood cell count: 32, 75.
Low white blood cell count: 32, 75, 24.
Low immunity: 24, 75, 79.
Low sperm count: 77, 78, 95, 96.
Low libido in men: 34, 78, 81, 94, 96, 98.
Low libido in women: 32, 81, 96, 98.
Lump in the throat: 27, 34.
Lumps in the breast: 26, 34, 90, 96.
Macular degeneration: 83, 91, 92.
Manic disorders: 31, 78, 90, 93, 95.
Mastitis: 23, 26, 45, 83, 89.
Menopausal disorders: 31, 32, 34, 36, 47, 76, 96, 98.
Mental disorders: 1, 15, 28, 46, 49, 58, 77, 83, 90, 100.
Mood swings: 34, 70, 78, 95.
Multiple sclerosis: 1, 15, 46, 51, 84, 85, 94, 95, 96.
Muscle spasm of the upper back: 54, 64, 65, 88, 89.
Muscular atrophy: 74, 86, 94, 92, 91, 85
Muscular dystrophy: 74, 85, 86, 92, 111.
Mutism: 16, 21, 22, 46, 49.
Myelitis: 43, 72, 75, 94.
Myopia: 13, 16.
Neck pains and stiffness: 4, 50, 62, 63, 99.
Neuroma: 85, 103.
Neurotic vomiting: 31, 46, 82.
Never happy with anything: 49, 70.
Night sweats: 49, 51, 54, 66, 94.
Night blindness: 91, 92.
Nocturnal emission: 39, 40, 72, 74, 82.
Pain in the face: 11, 13.
Pain around the umbilicus: 31, 36, 38.
Pain behind the ear: 7, 8, 9, 47, 61, 63.
Pain in the hypochondriac region: 23, 49, 85, 89.
Pain in the external genitalia (Groin): 15, 46, 49, 78, 81, 95, 96, 106.
Pain in the heel: 98, 99, 100.
Pain and motor impairment of the shoulder: 23, 68, 88.
Pain in the testicles: 15, 46, 49, 79, 89
Pain of the dorsum of the foot: 97, 98, 99, 103.
Pain in the scapula (Upper back): 54, 67, 88, 95, 96.

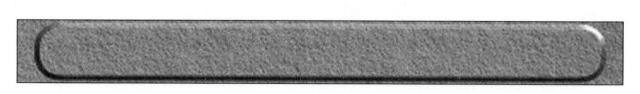

Pain in the lateral (outside) part of the upper arm: 23, 42, 44, 46.
Pain and stiffness of the lower back: 15, 76, 79.
Painful intercourse: 40, 75, 76, 78, 81, 96.
Paralysis of the foot: 1, 15, 94, 97, 98, 99, 102.
Paralysis of the limbs: 1, 15, 50, 51, 85, 92, 94, 97, 98, 99, 102.
Phobias: 46, 49, 50, 52, 63.
Poor digestion of carbohydrates: 31, 83, 96.
Postnasal drips: 14, 25.
Prevent sagging breast: 23.
Prevent sleeping: 42.
Promote yawning: 46, 50, 51, 95.
Pruritus vulvae: 78, 96, 100.
Psoriasis: 31, 46, 78, 95.
Reduce fat from the thighs: 16, 85.
Sensation of plugged ears: 47, 93.
Spontaneous sweating: 49, 94.
Sprain ankle: 97, 98, 99, 103.
Stage fright: 19, 21, 22, 46, 49, 70.
Sterility in women: 78, 96, 111.
Sugar craving: 31, 44, 46, 49, 83, 96.
T.M.J. pain: 7, 8, 9, 11, 46, 53.
Tearing of the eyes: 5, 6, 12.
Temper tantrum in children: 44, 46, 49, 106.
To increase bust size in women: 23.
To decrease appetite: 46, 49.
To calm down: 46, 52.
To mend broken hearts: 49.
To reduce wrinkles: 98.
To boost up energy: 83.
Too much sweating: 78.
Tunnel vision: 91, 92.
Twitching of any part of the body: 34, 35.
Twitching of the eyelids: 4, 8, 12, 13, 16, 31, 34, 35, 54.
Unhappy disposition: 11, 46, 49, 52, 65, 69.
Varicose veins: 52, 80, 96.
Vertigo: 1, 34, 100.
Warts: 31, 95, 96.

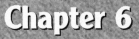
Points with
Illustrations

POINTS: 38, 39, 53, 83, 87, 97, 102.

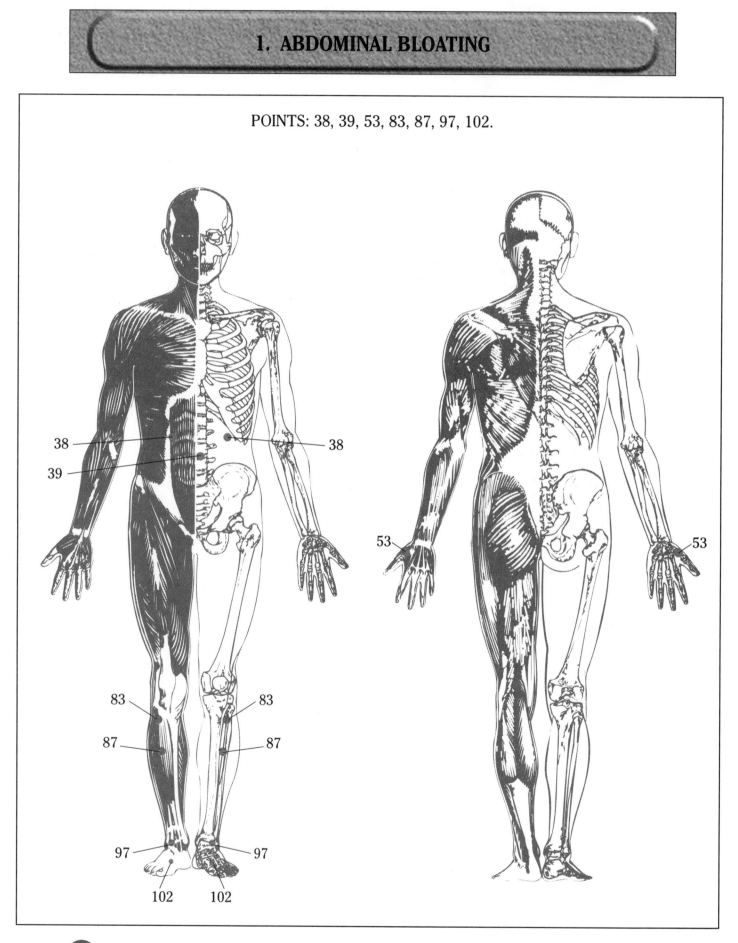

2. ABDOMINAL PAIN

POINTS: 15, 31, 38, 39, 46, 53, 83, 82, 87, 89, 103

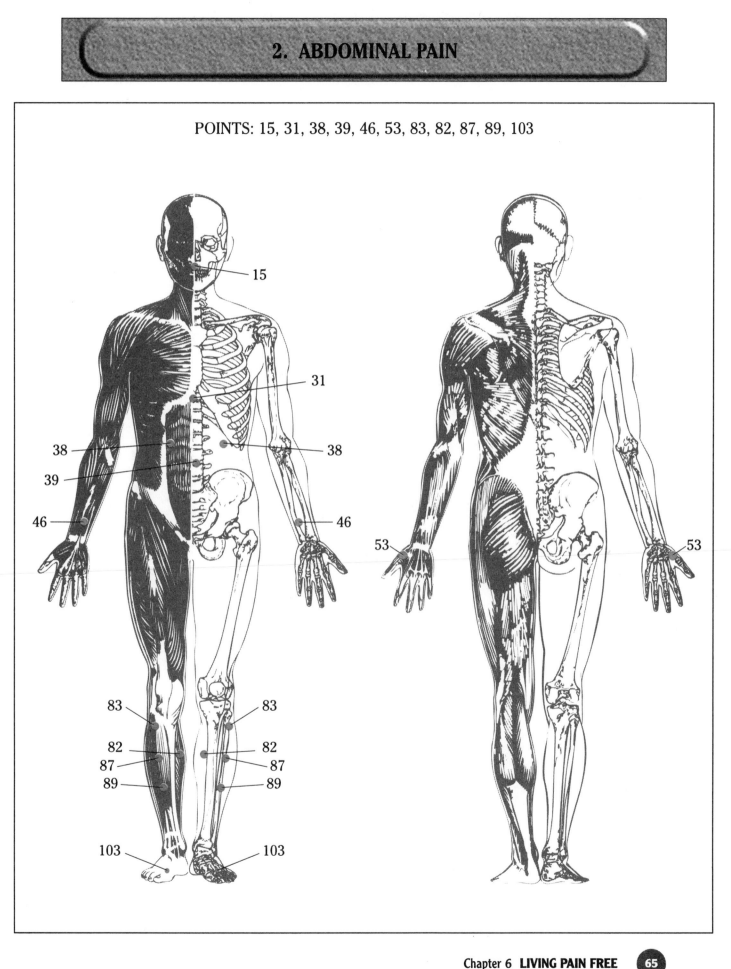

POINTS: 31, 57, 83, 103, 108.

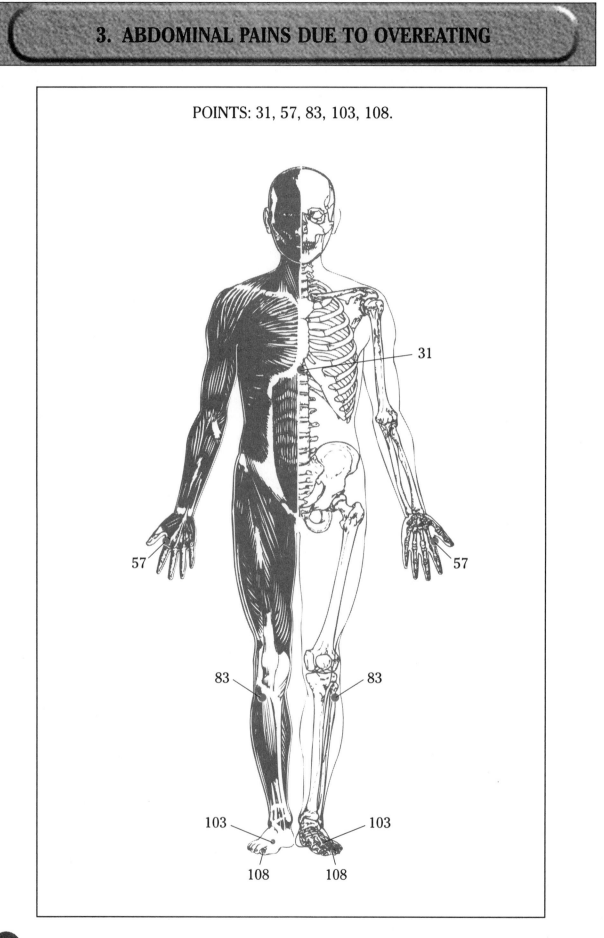

4. ABDOMINAL SPASMS

POINTS: 36, 40, 41, 42, 57, 71, 84, 103.

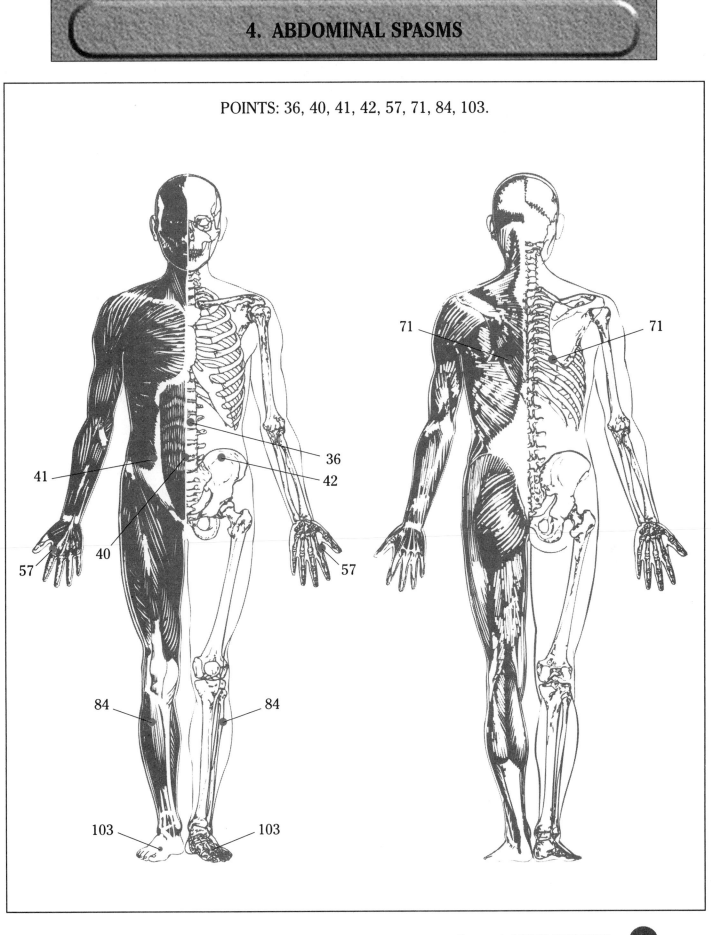

POINTS: 40, 53, 57, 87, 96.

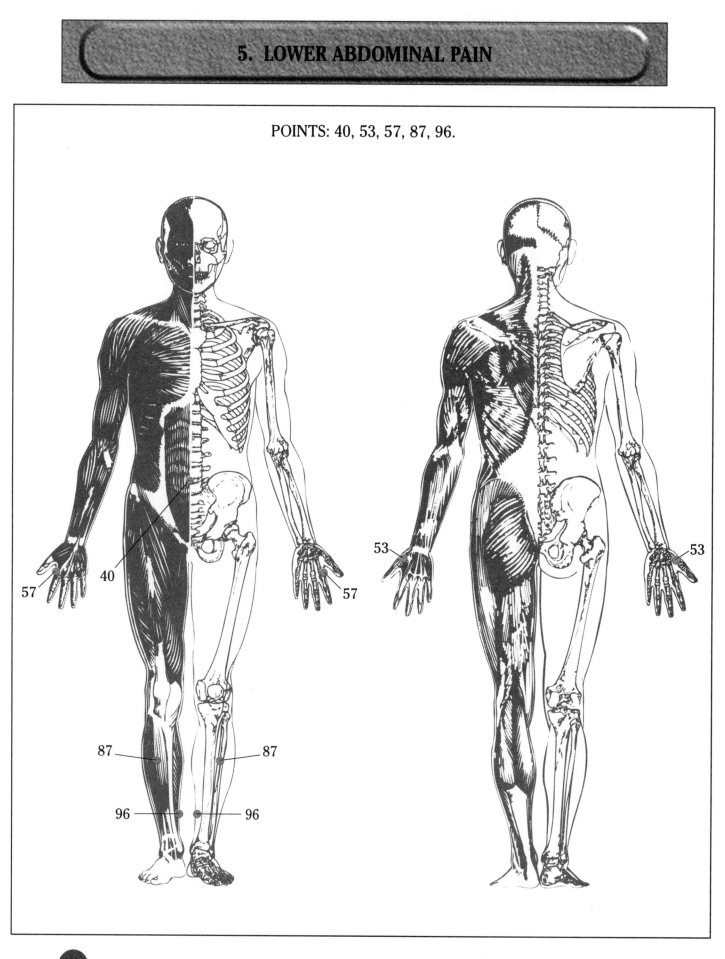

POINTS: 14, 24, 25, 31, 44, 63, 75, 79.

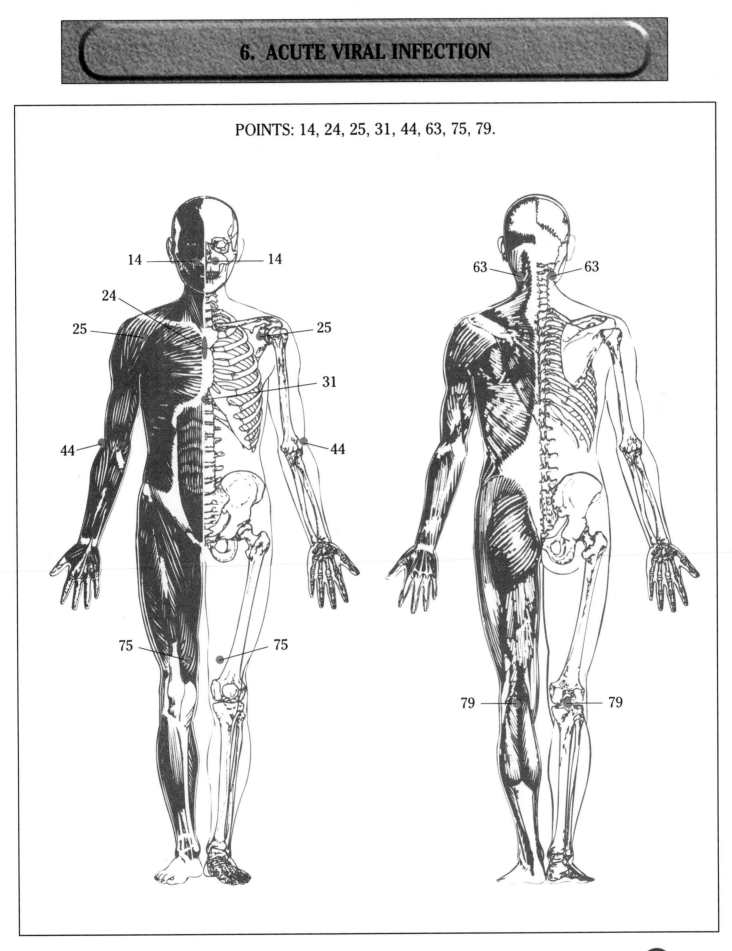

POINTS: 15, 53, 57, 83, 84, 87.

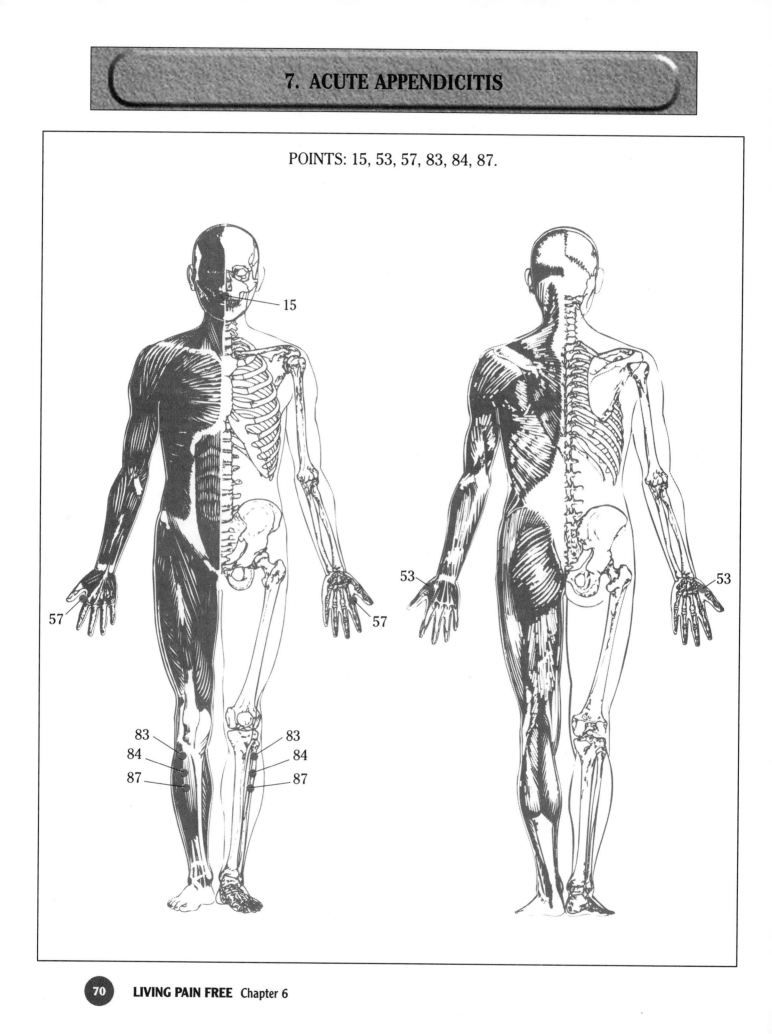

POINTS: 5, 31, 32, 34, 44, 46, 49, 22.

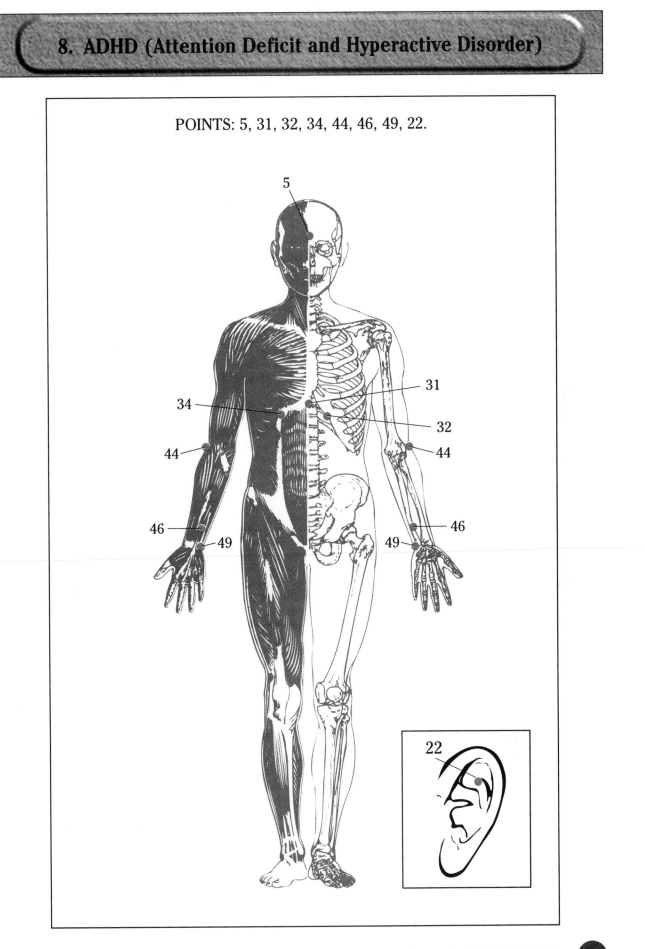

9. ACNE

POINTS: 37, 42, 44, 75, 87.

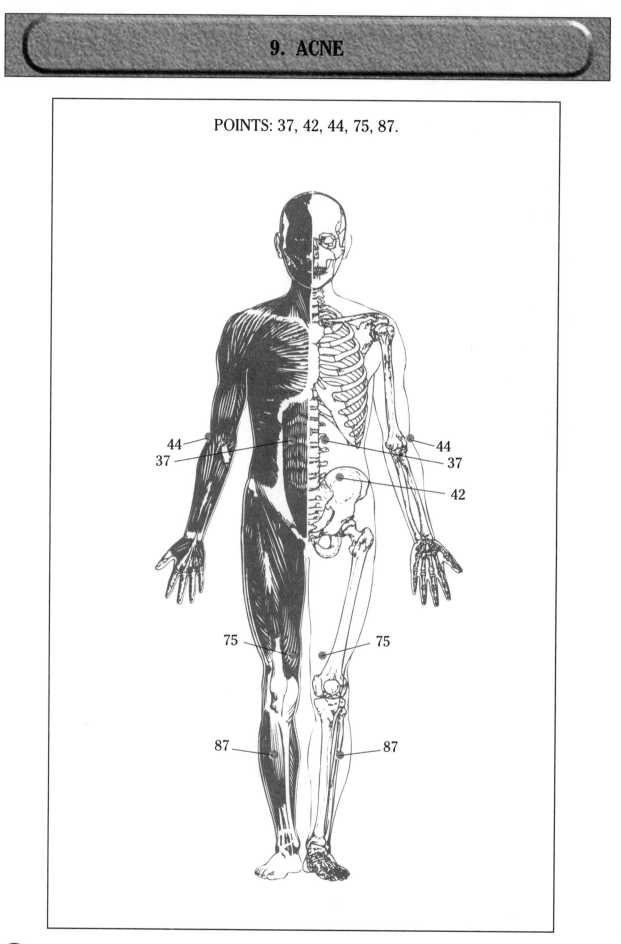

POINTS: 5, 22, 31, 32, 34, 44, 46, 49.

ADDICTION TO FOOD
ADDICTION TO DRUGS
ADDICTION TO CAFFEINE
ADDICTION TO CHOCOLATE
ADDICTION TO ALCOHOL

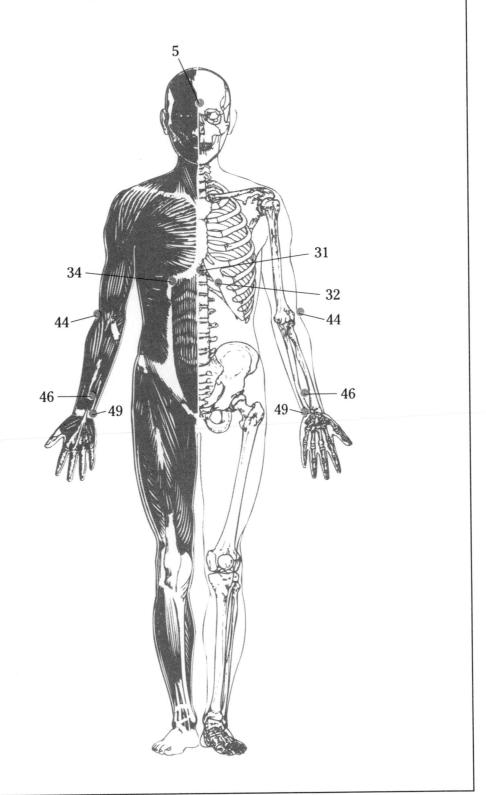

POINTS: 22, 34, 44, 46, 49, 52, 102.

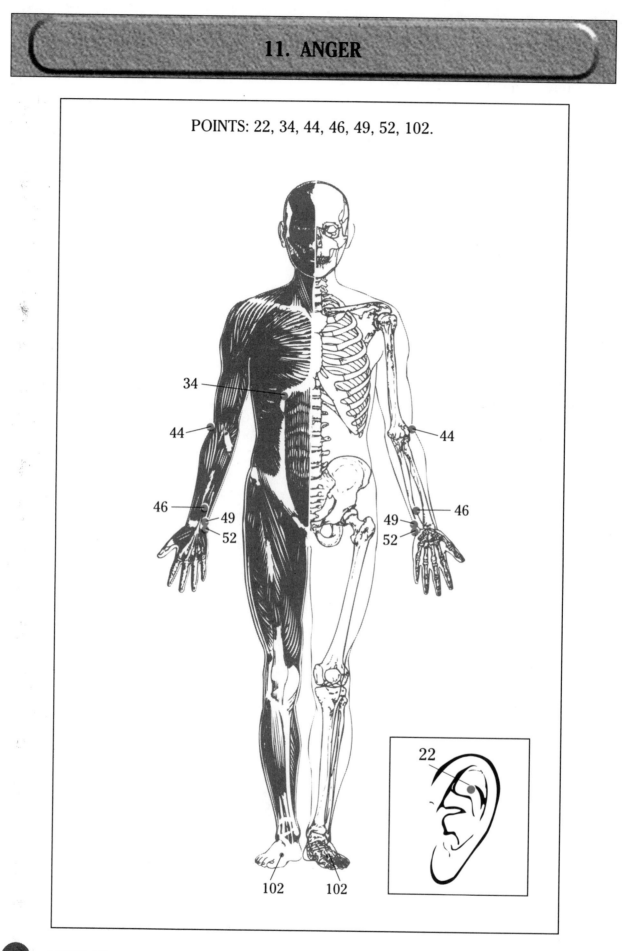

12. ANGIONEUROTIC EDEMA

POINTS: 24, 25R, 25L, 31, 44, 46, 61, 81, 93.

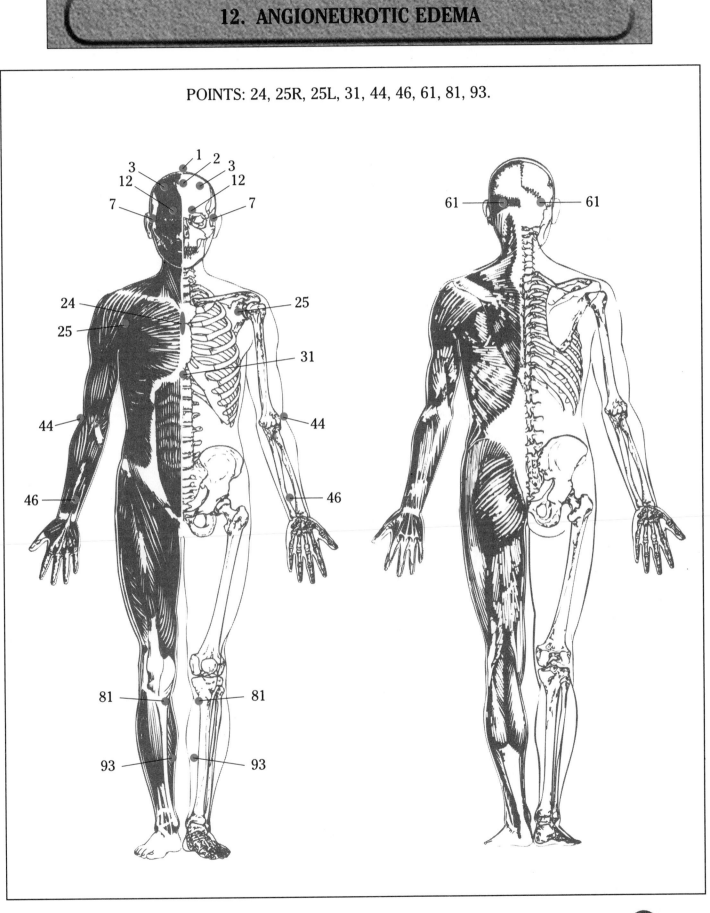

POINTS: 31, 46, 49, 52, 82.

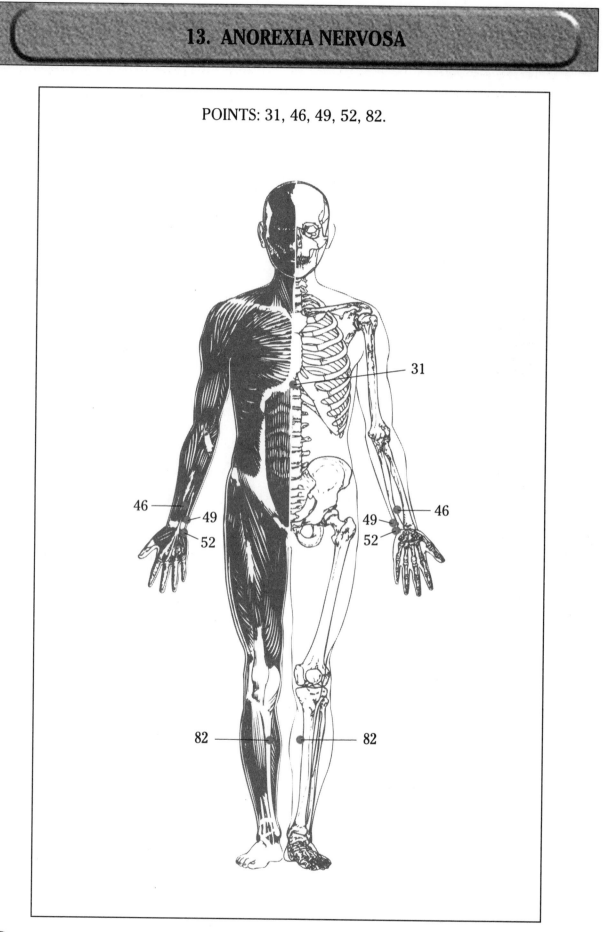

14. ANXIETY ATTACKS

POINTS: 2, 69, 78, 98, 101, 106.

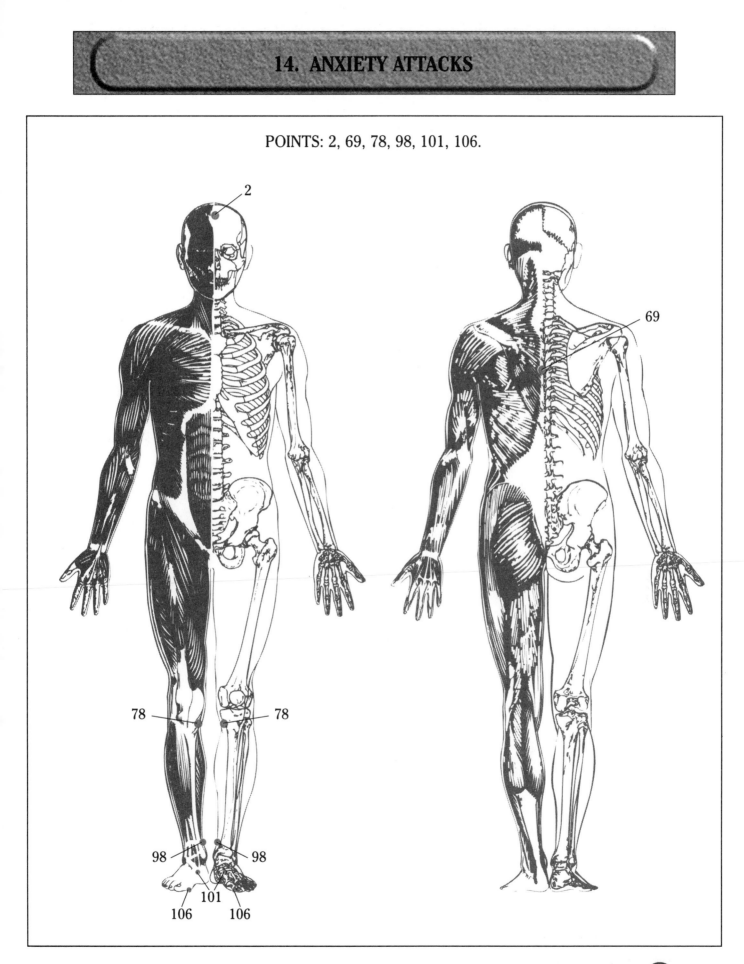

15. ARTHRITIS OF THE FINGERS

POINTS: 32, 33, 46, 49, 52.

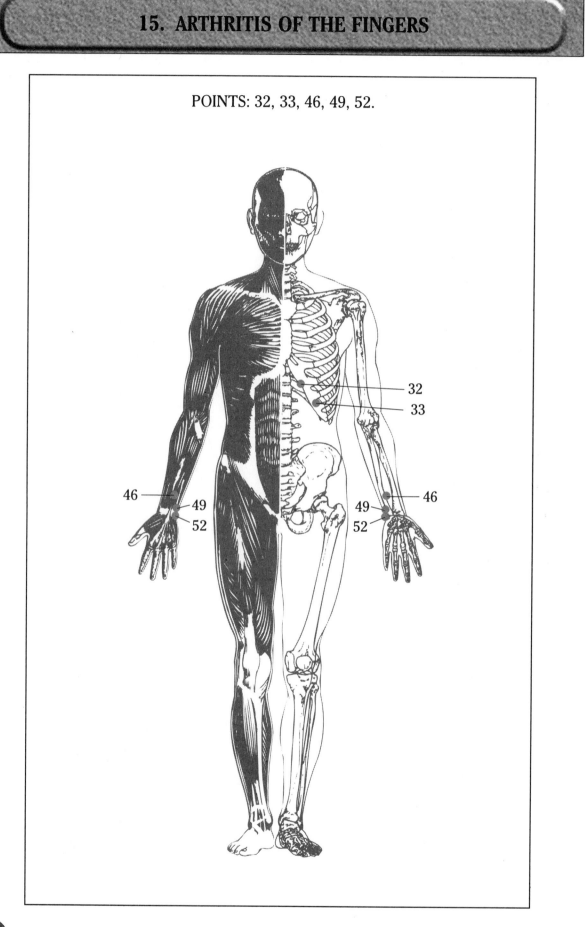

POINTS: 46, 47, 48, 49.

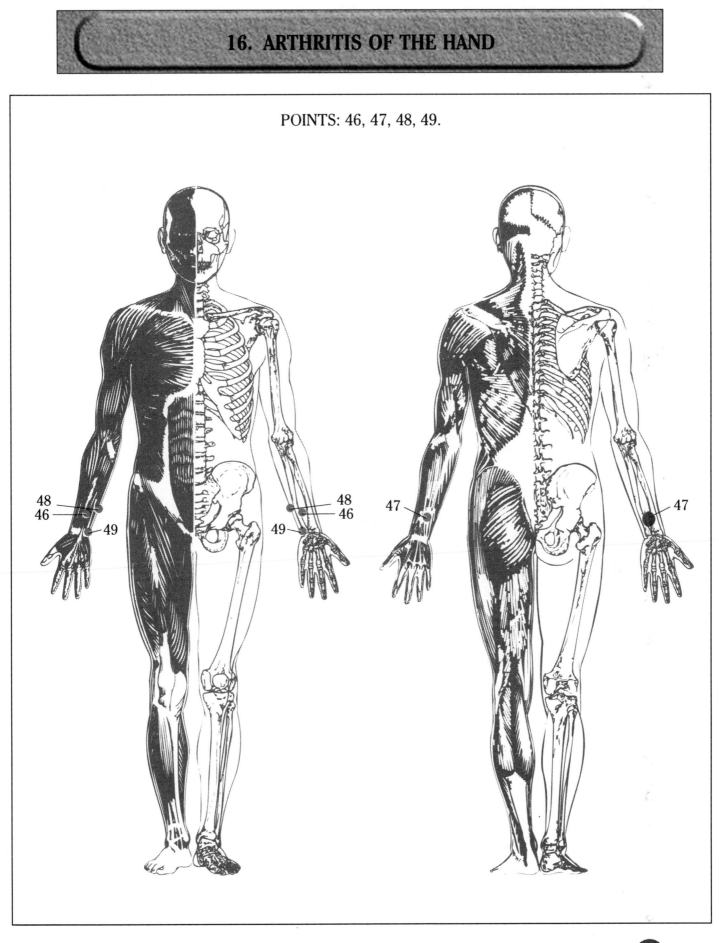

POINTS: 23, 38, 44, 45, 46, 87.

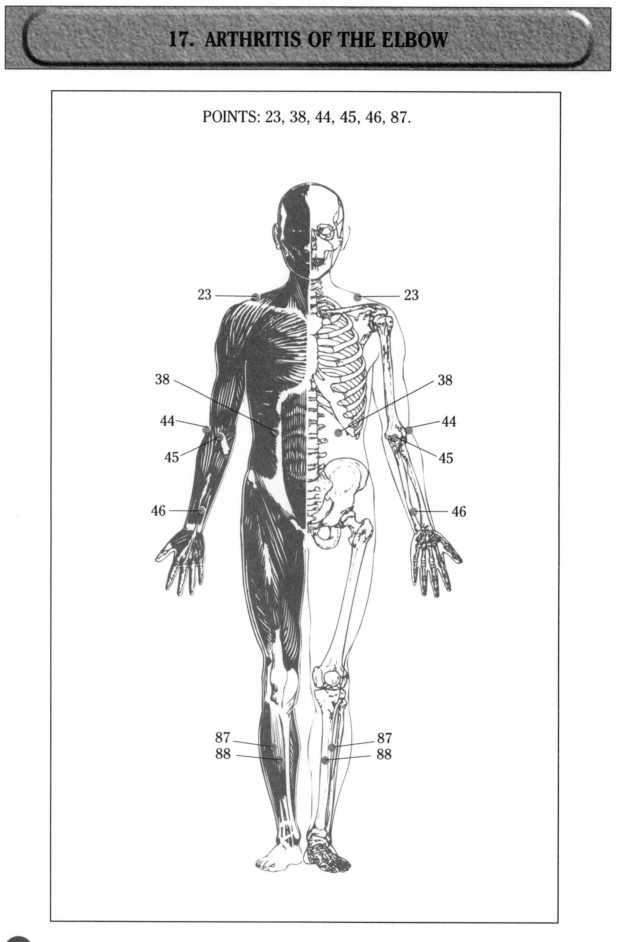

18. ARTHRITIS OF THE SHOULDER

POINTS: 23, 25, 32, 67, 68, 88.

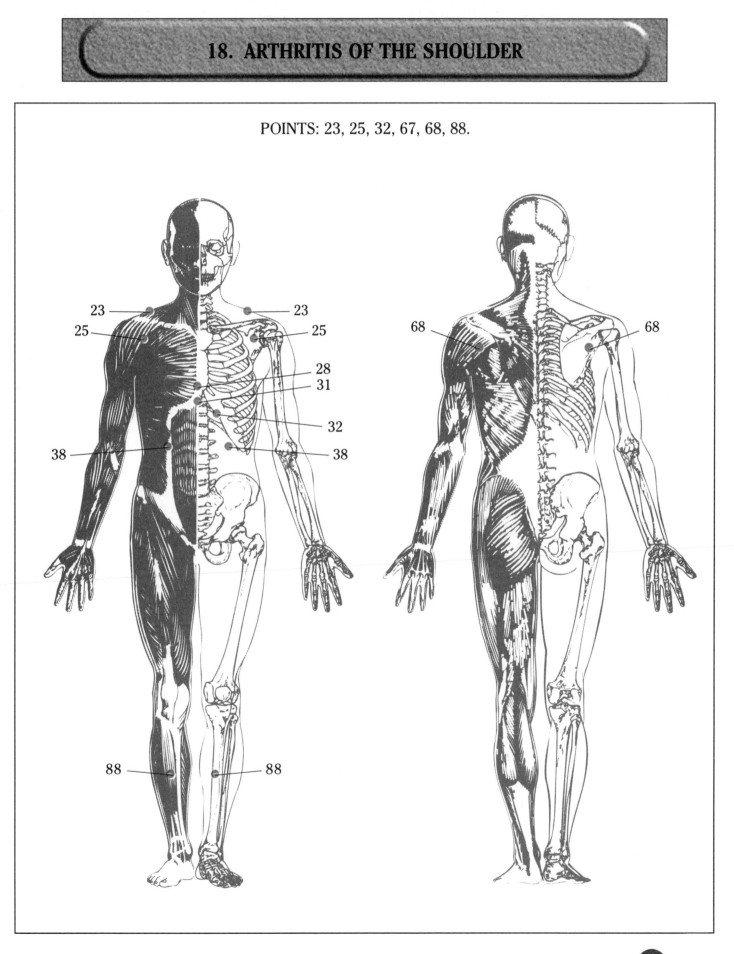

POINTS: 43, 46, 47, 49, 53, 54.

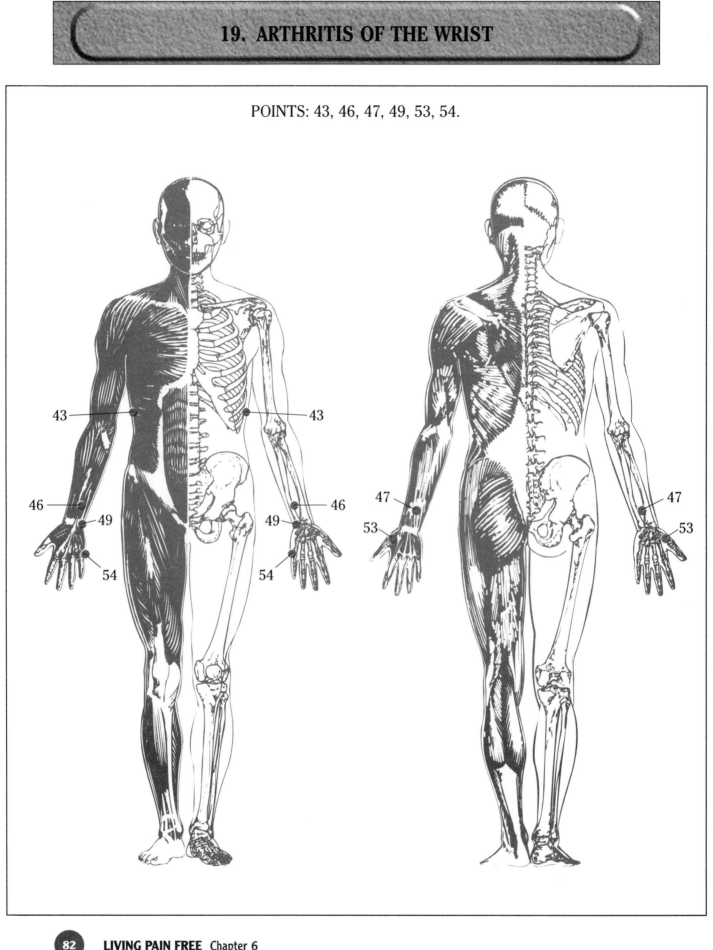

20. ARTHRITIS OF THE HIP JOINT

POINTS: 41, 42, 40, 43, 46, 77, 74, 87.

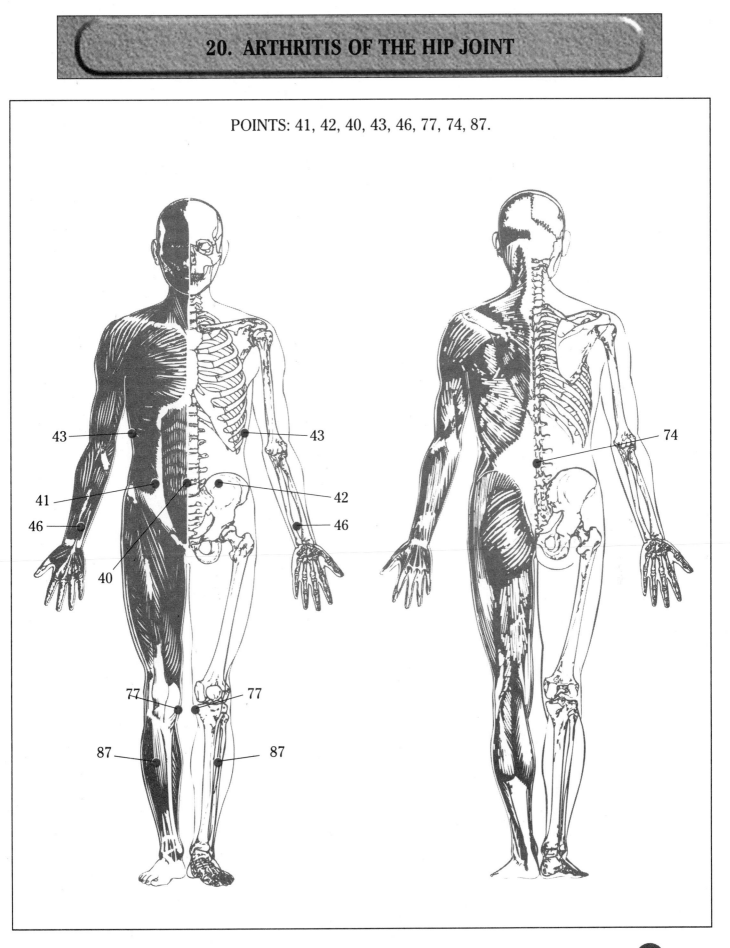

21. ARTHRITIS OF THE KNEE

POINTS: 75, 76, 78, 79, 81, 83, 87.

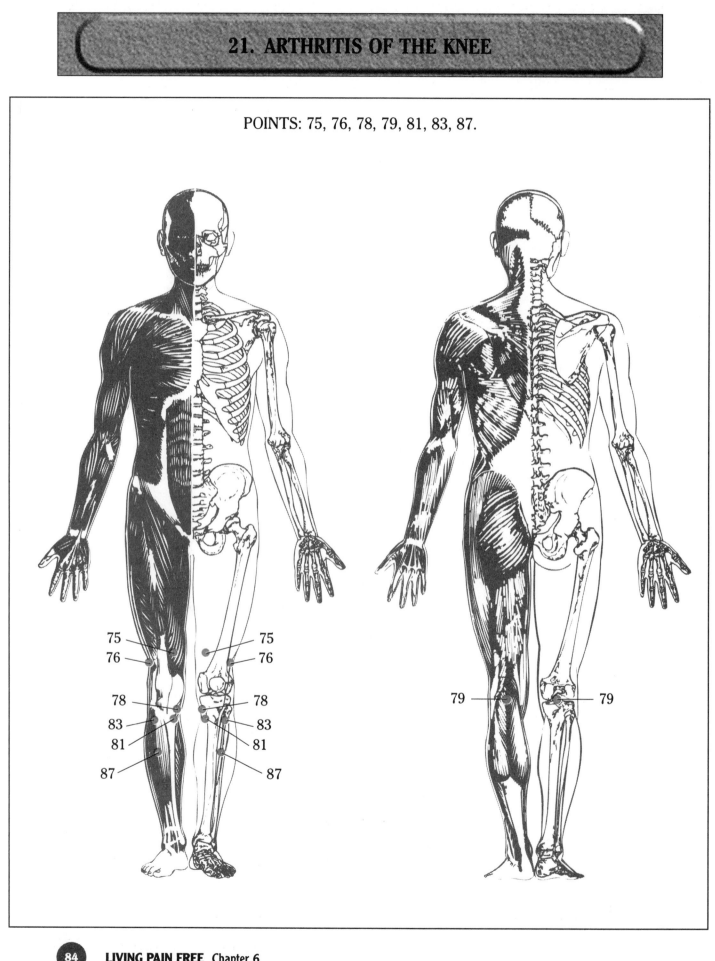

POINTS: 77, 78, 81, 96, 98, 99, 103, 104.

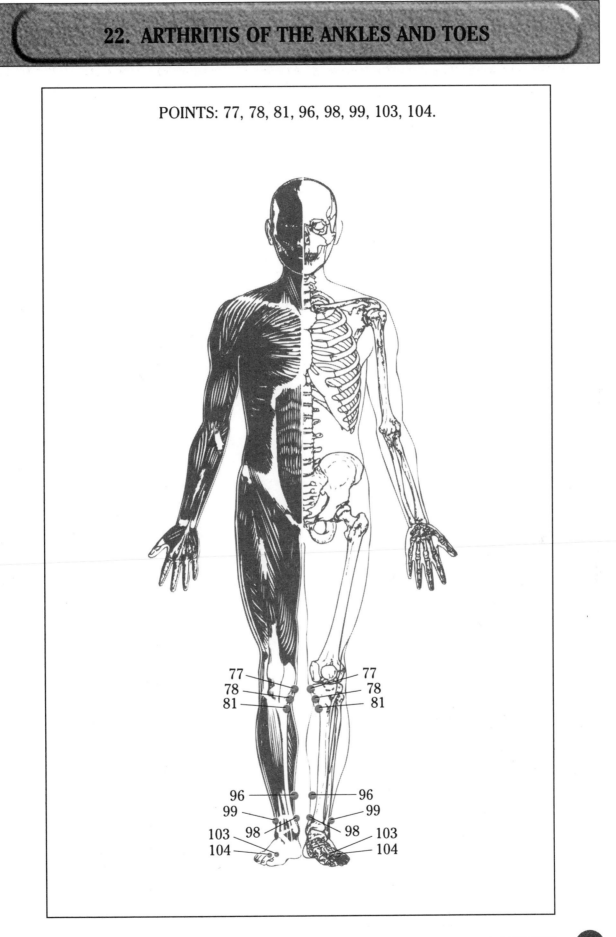

POINTS: 15, 30, 44, 53, 54, 75, 83, 107.

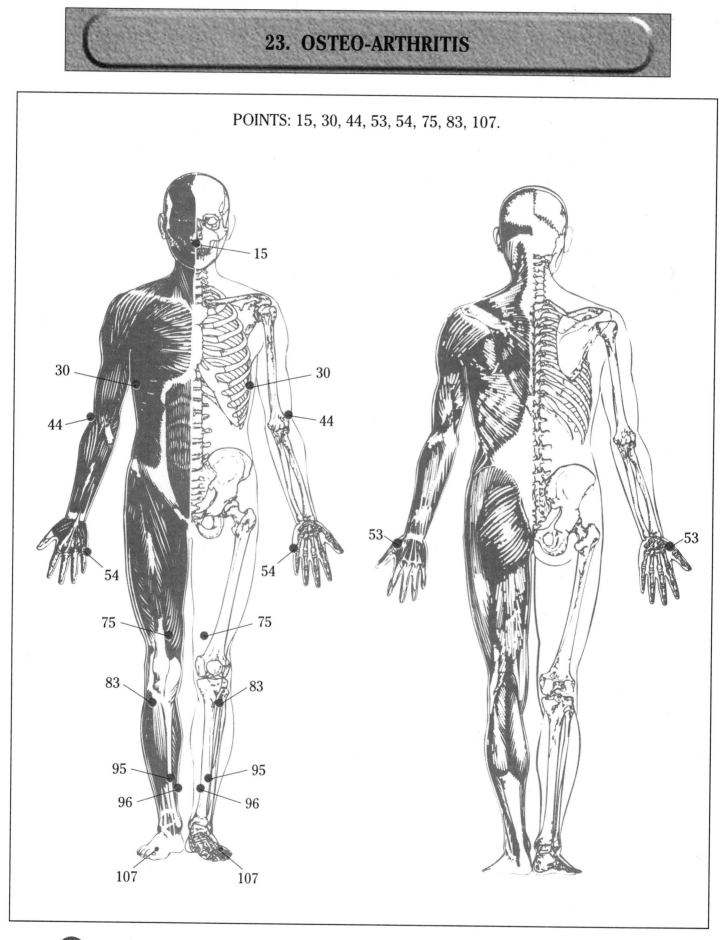

24. RHEUMATOID-ARTHRITIS

POINTS: 15, 30, 44, 53, 54, 75, 95, 96, 101, 107.

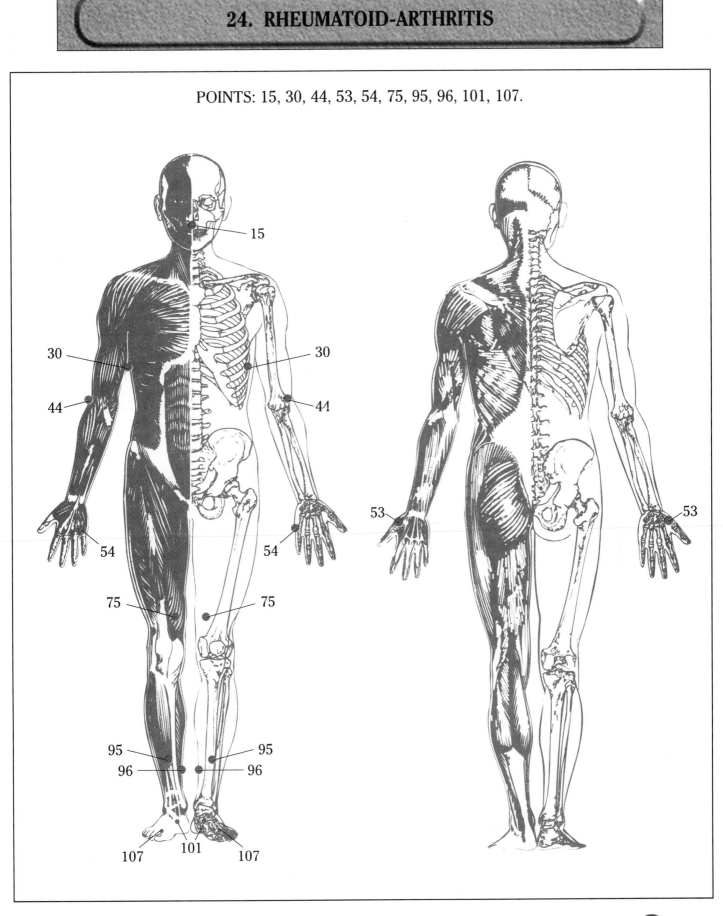

POINTS: 15, 30, 44, 53, 54, 75, 85, 95, 96, 101, 102.

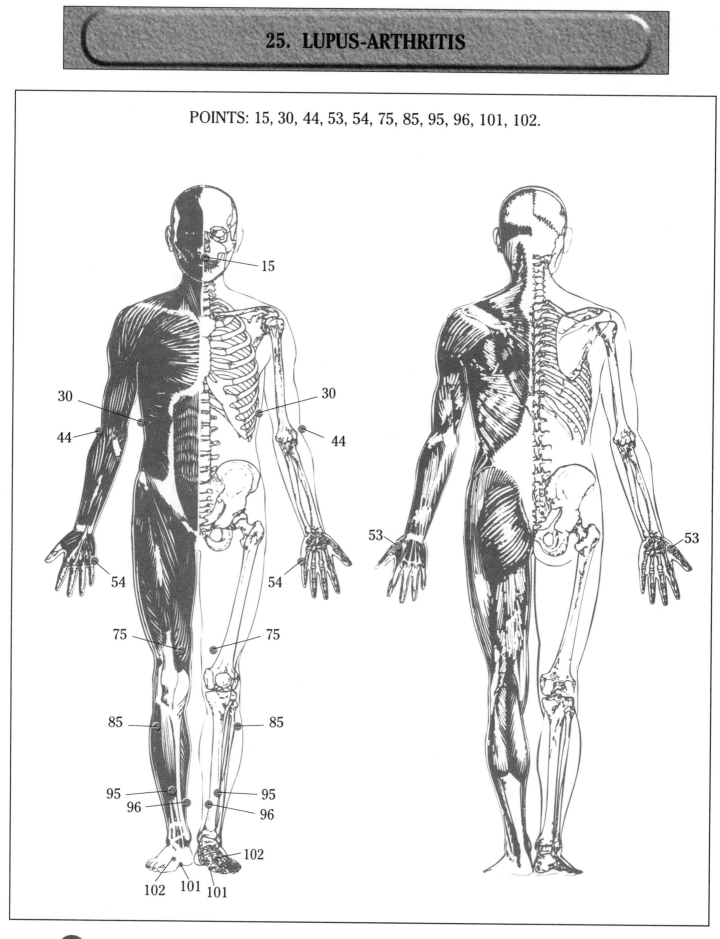

POINTS: 38, 81, 90, 101.

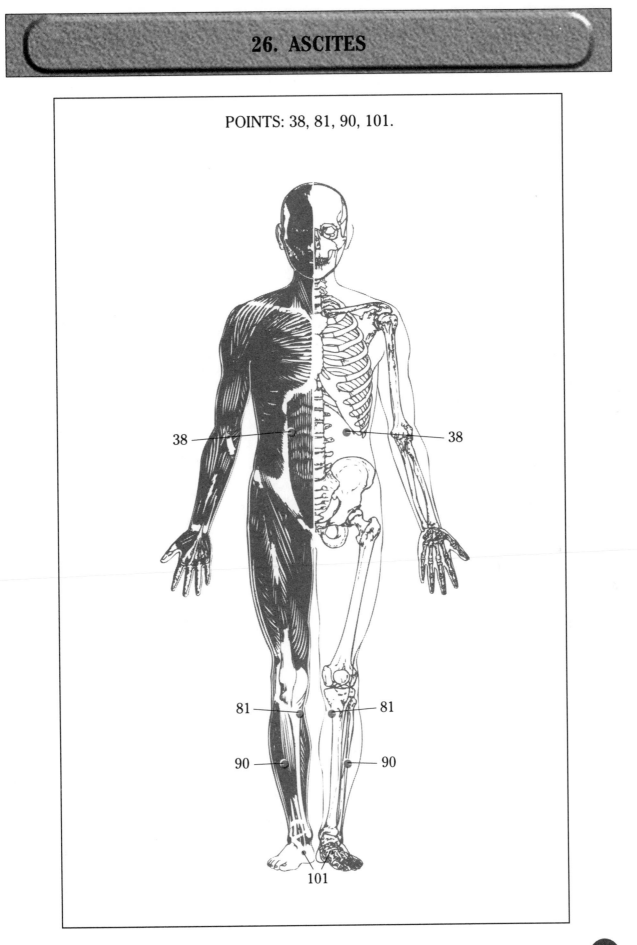

POINTS: 20, 25, 26, 28, 39, 45, 50, 64, 65, 66, 90, 98.

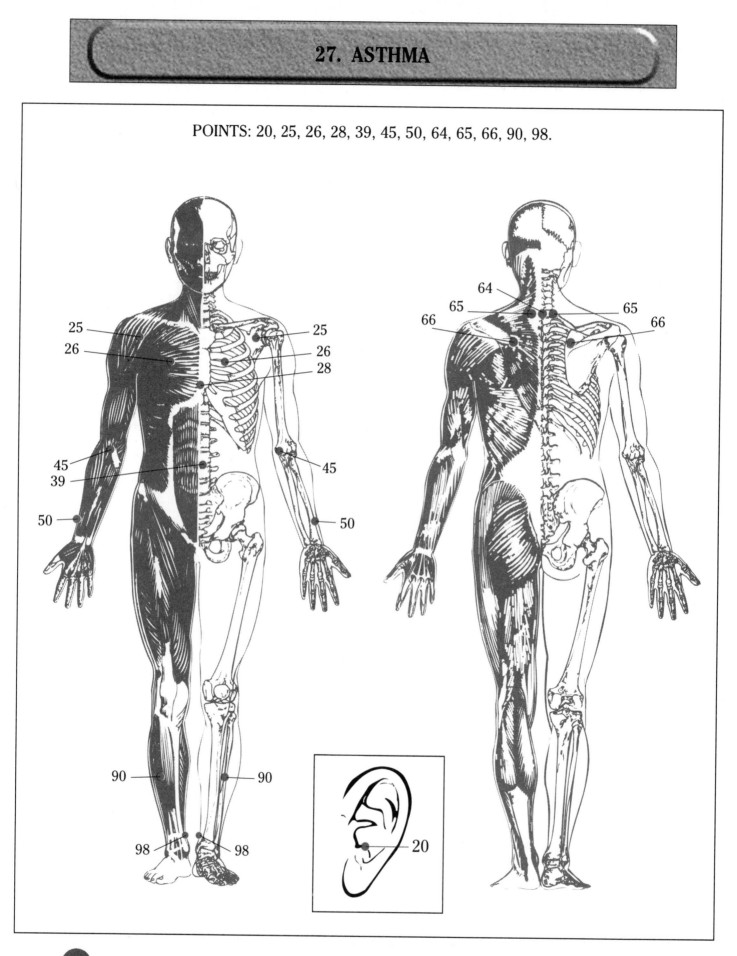

POINTS: 15, 46, 57, 72, 74, 79.

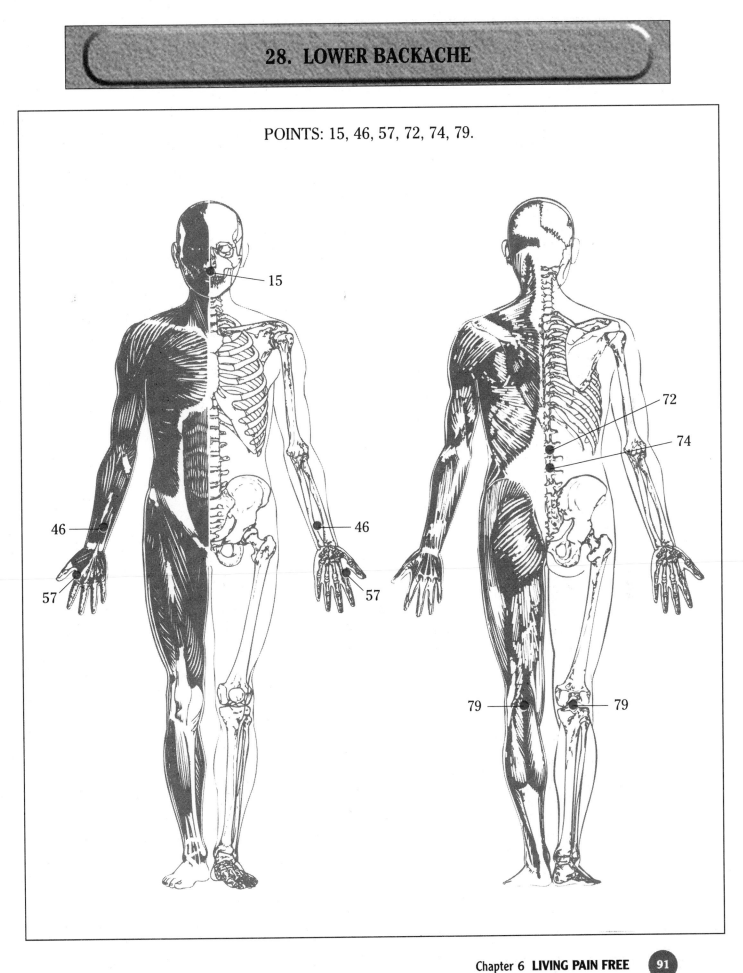

29. MID BACKACHE

POINTS: 30, 31, 32, 33, 34, 43, 46, 71, 83.

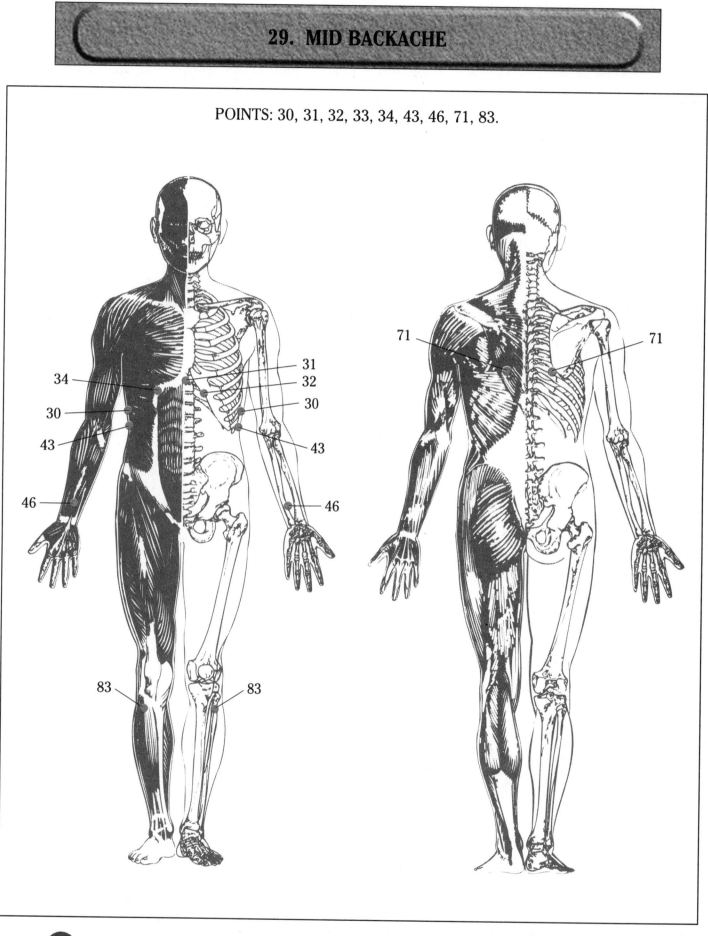

30. UPPER BACKACHE

POINTS: 23, 47, 54, 63, 64.

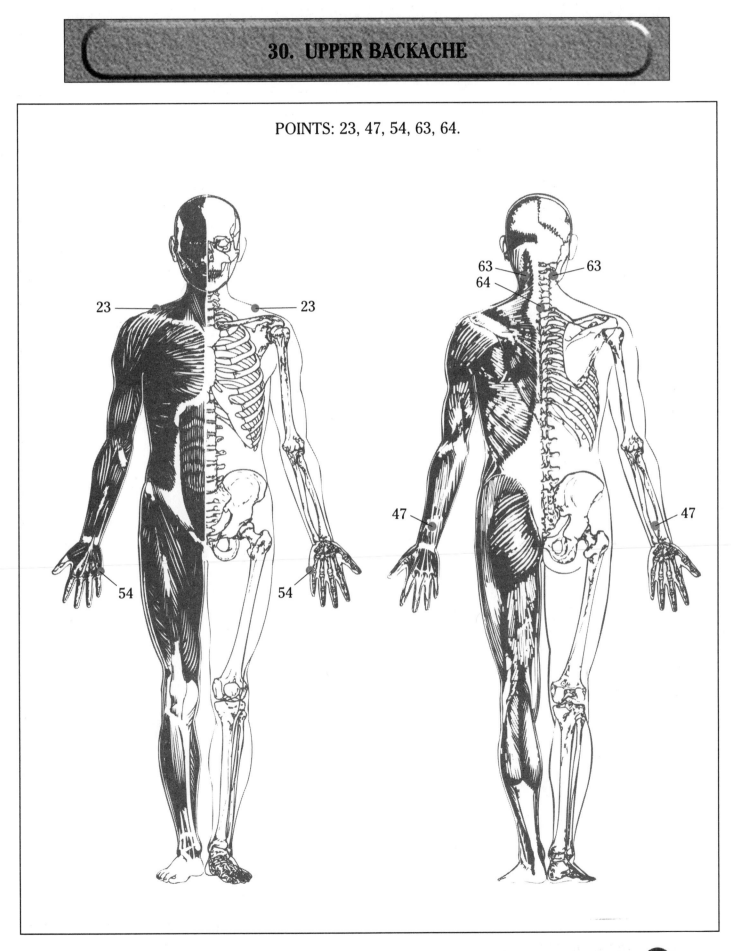

31. BACTERIAL INFECTION

POINTS: 24, 44, 75, 79.

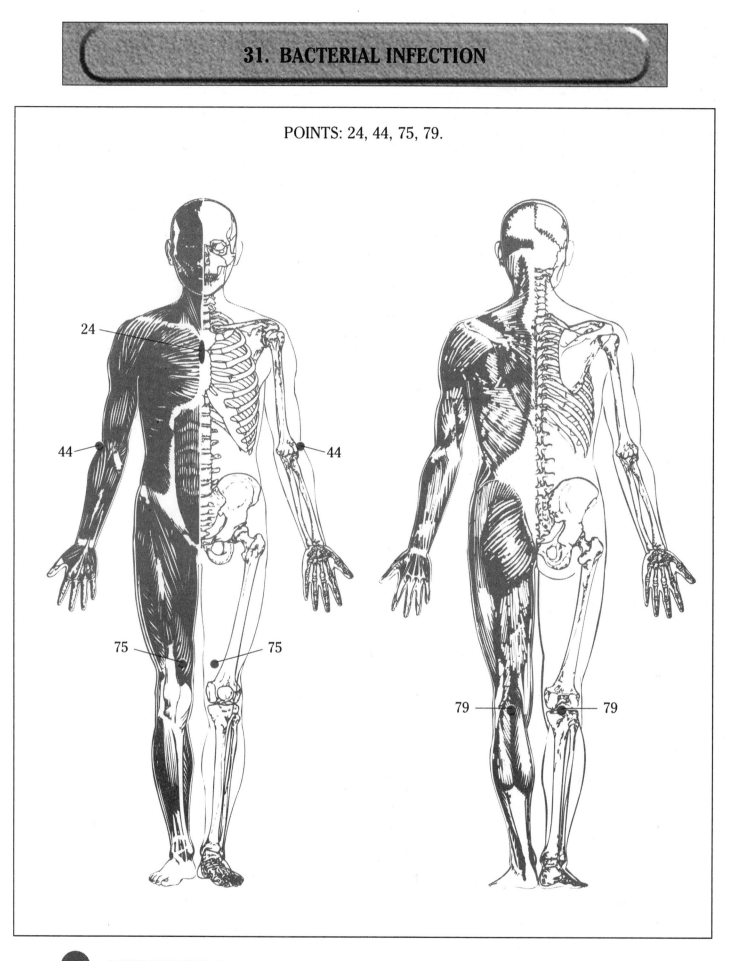

POINTS: 24, 31, 32, 51, 75, 102.

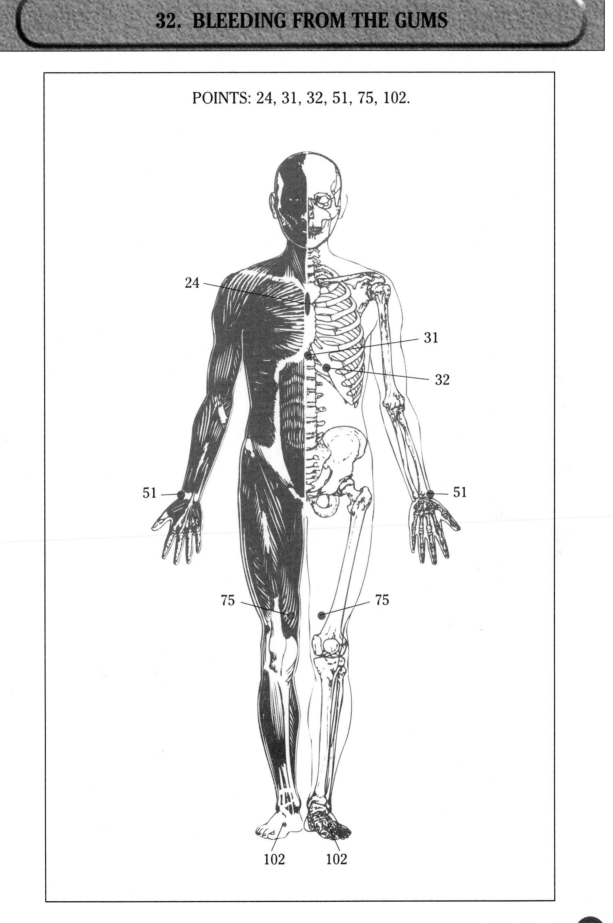

POINTS: 14, 34, 46, 97, 98, 99.

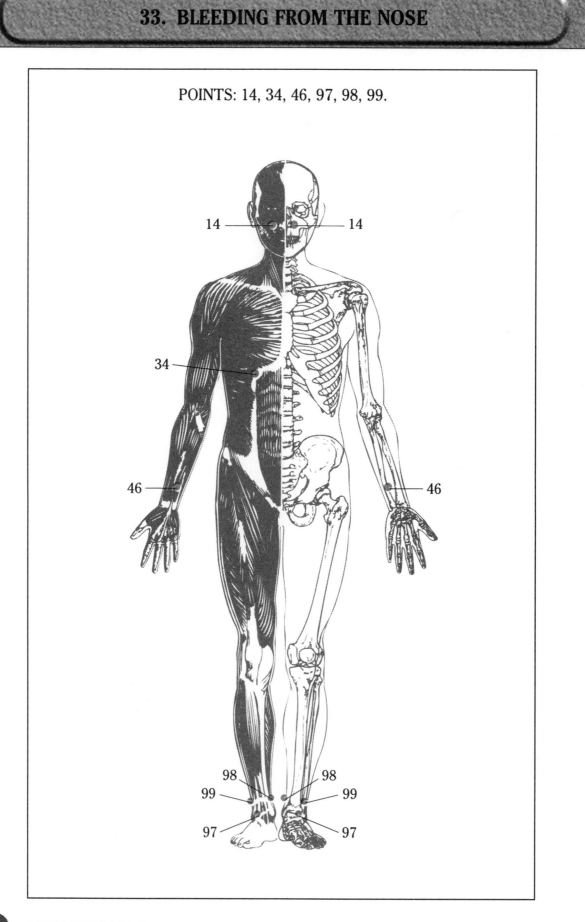

POINTS: 24, 34, 51, 75, 102.

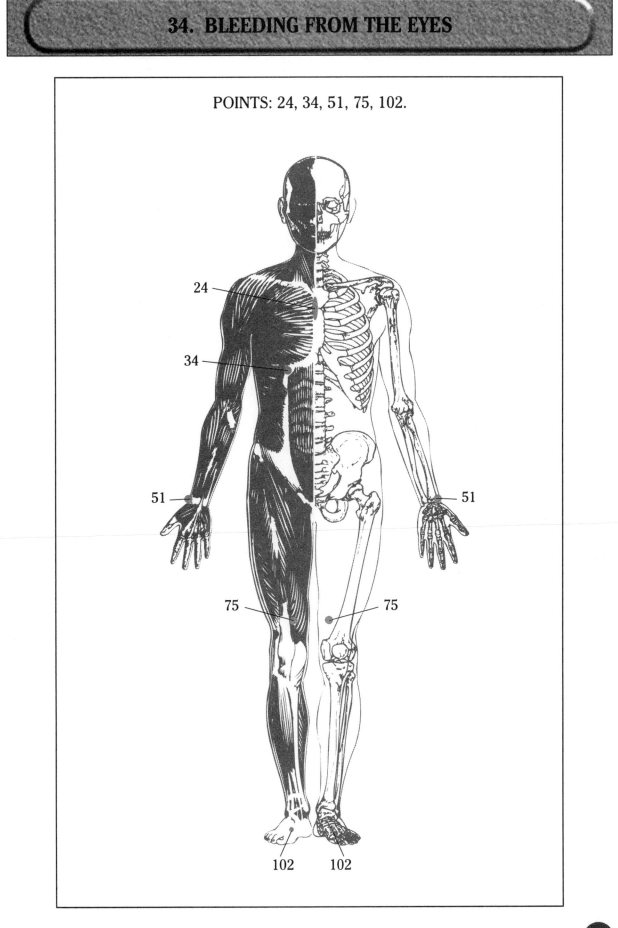

POINTS: 24, 46, 51, 57, 75, 102.

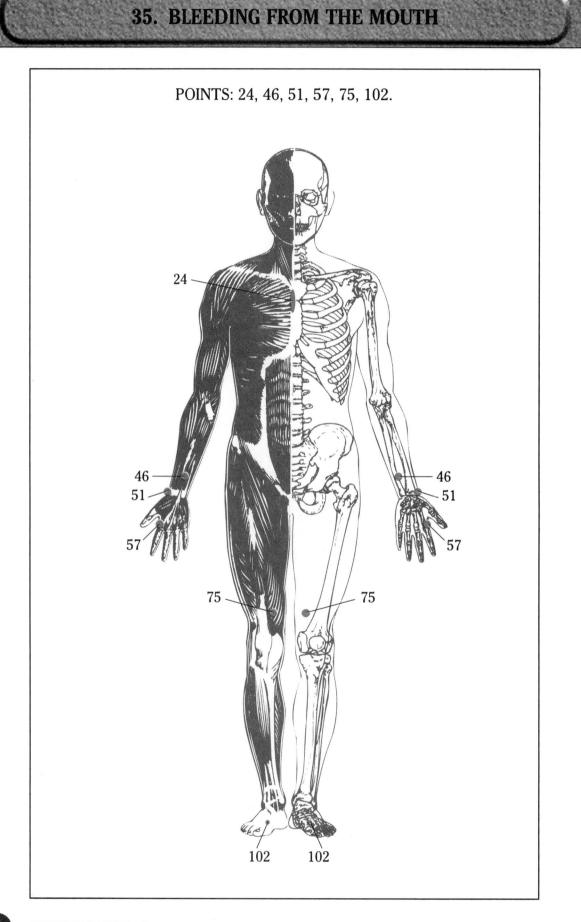

POINTS: 24, 32, 49, 51, 75, 102.

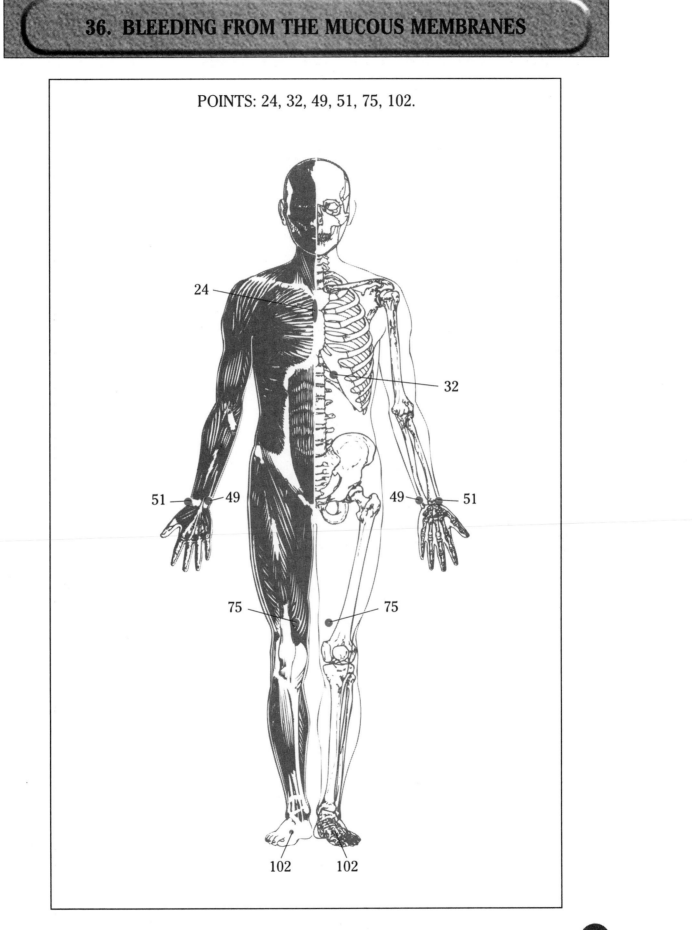

POINTS: 24, 31, 51, 75, 102.

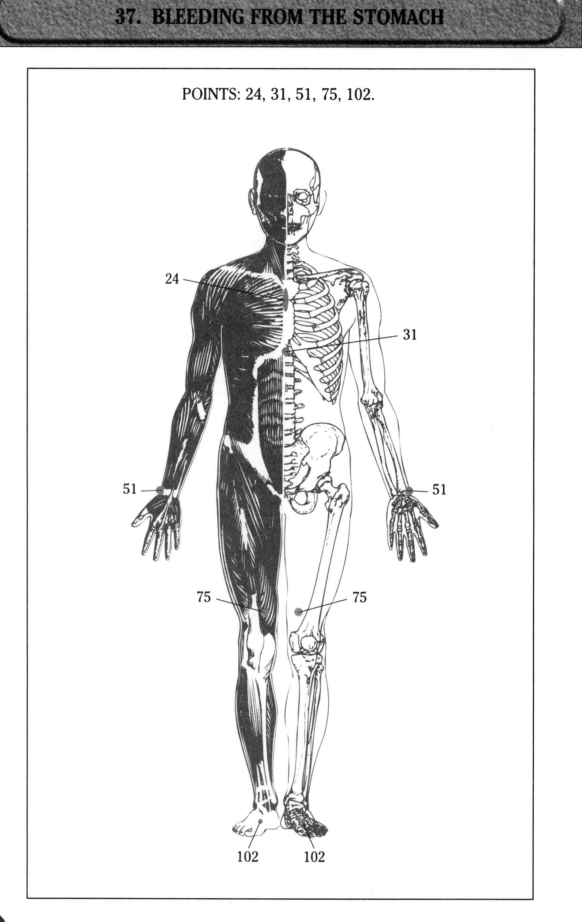

POINTS: 24, 32, 51, 66, 75, 82.

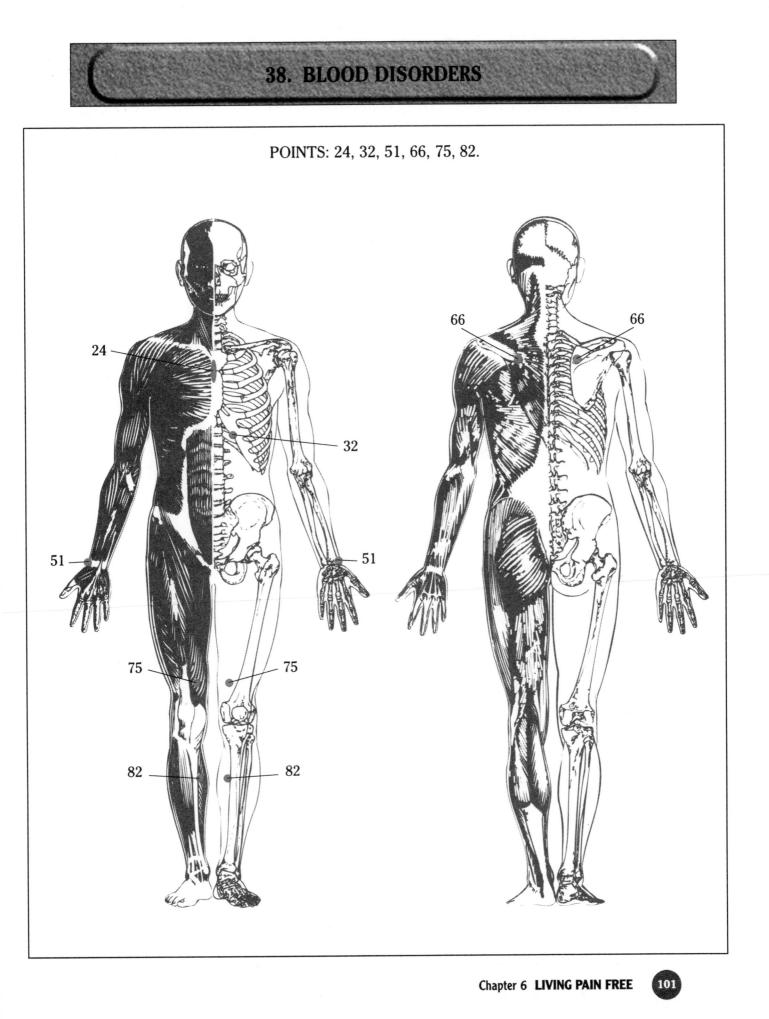

POINTS: 37, 87, 101, 106.

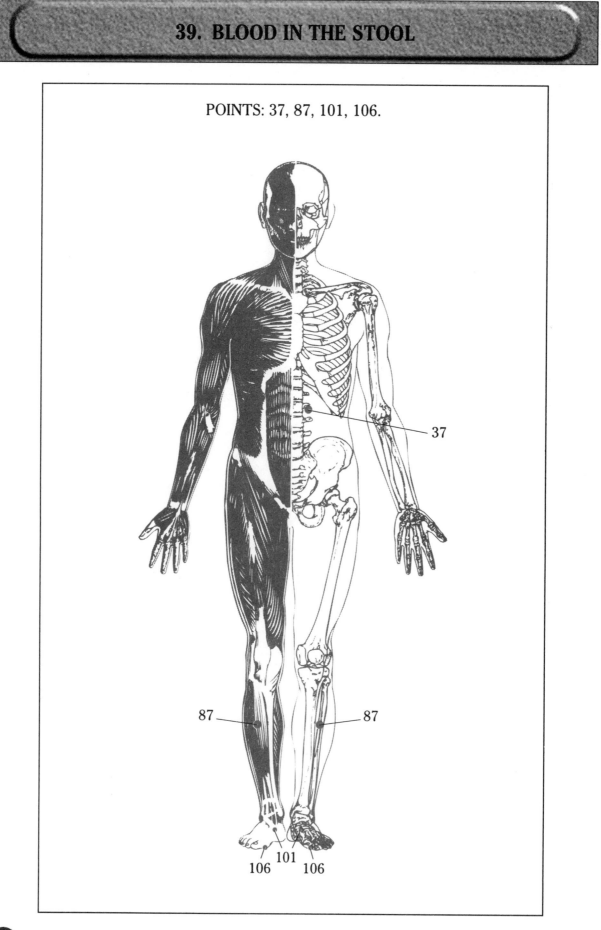

40. BLOOD IN THE URINE

POINTS: 37, 40, 75, 99, 106.

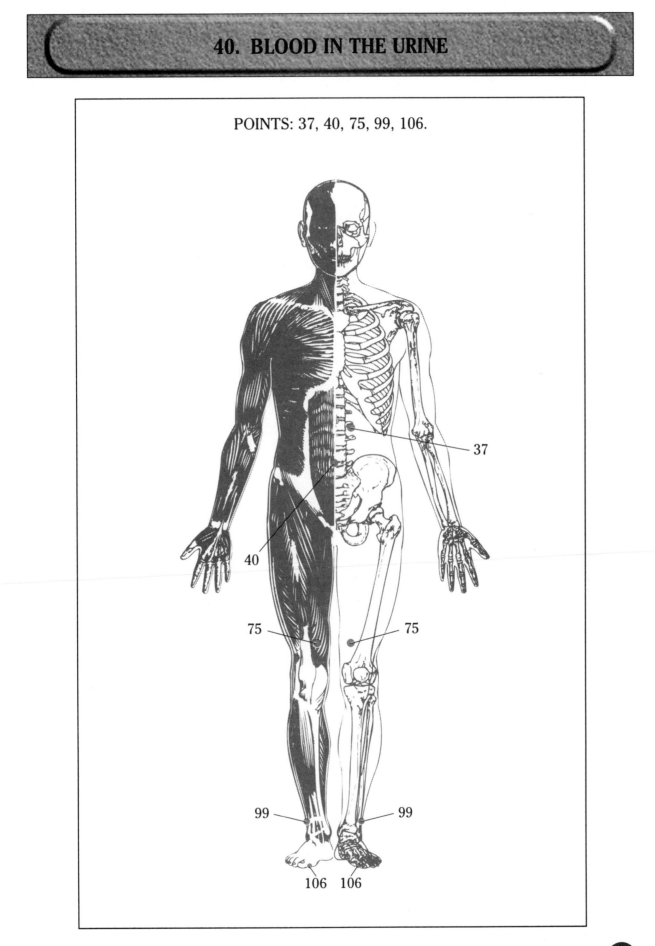

POINTS: 40, 82, 101, 107, 106.

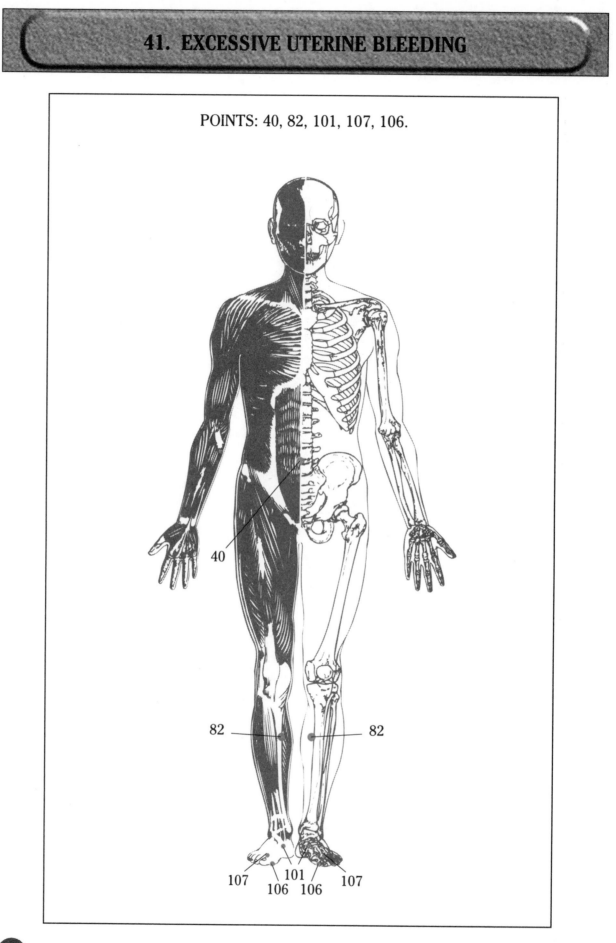

POINTS: 46, 82, 87, 101, 106, 107.

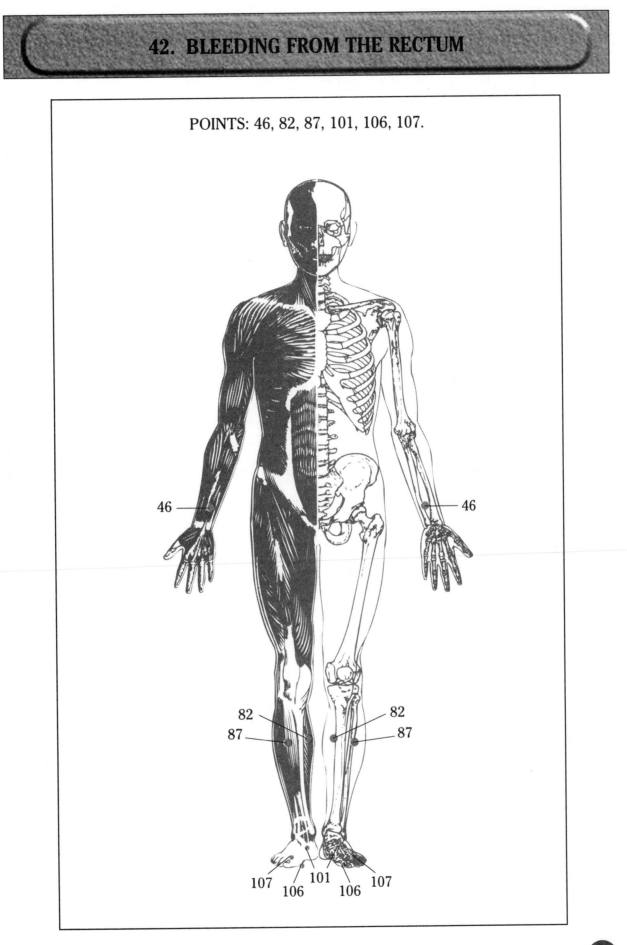

43. HEMORRHOIDS, BLEEDING OR IRRITATION

POINTS: 51, 57, 80, 82, 96, 97, 99.

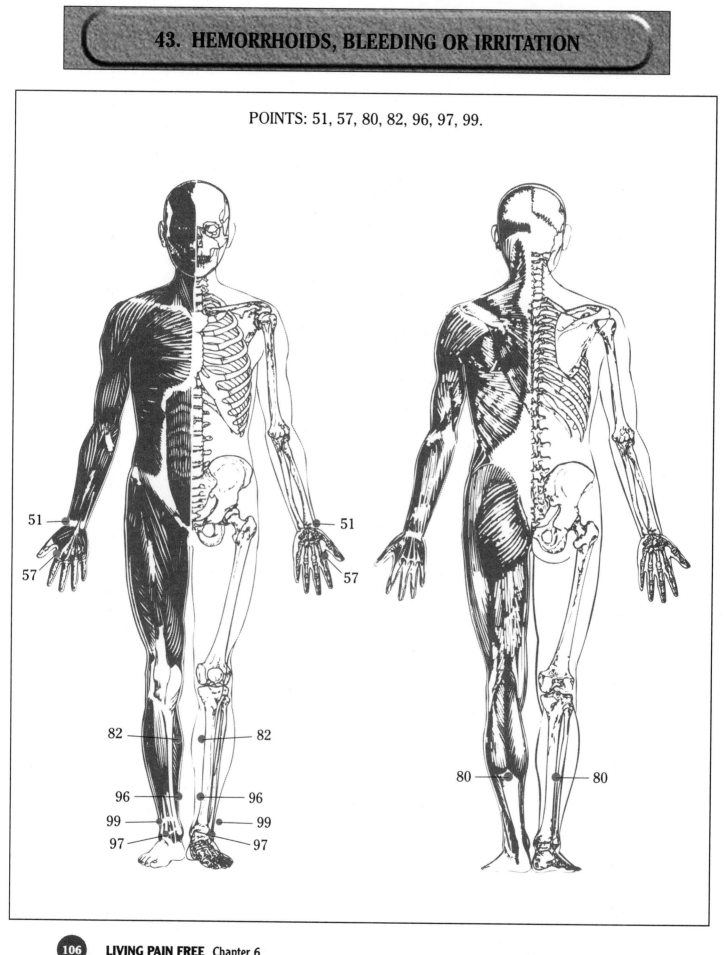

POINTS: 83, 94, 96, 98, 99, 101.

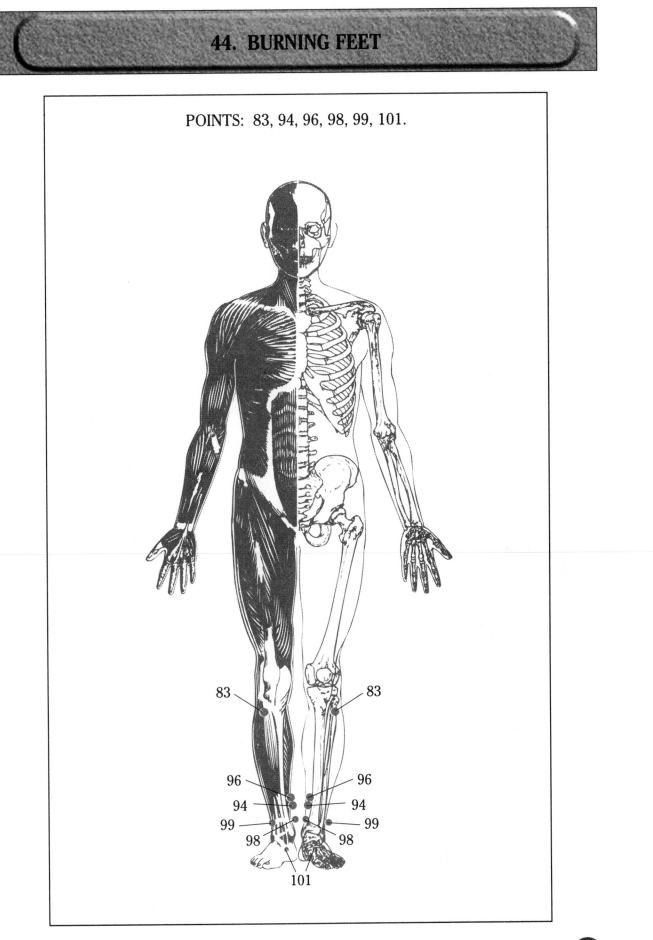

POINTS: 1, 2, 12, 13, 14, 53, 65.

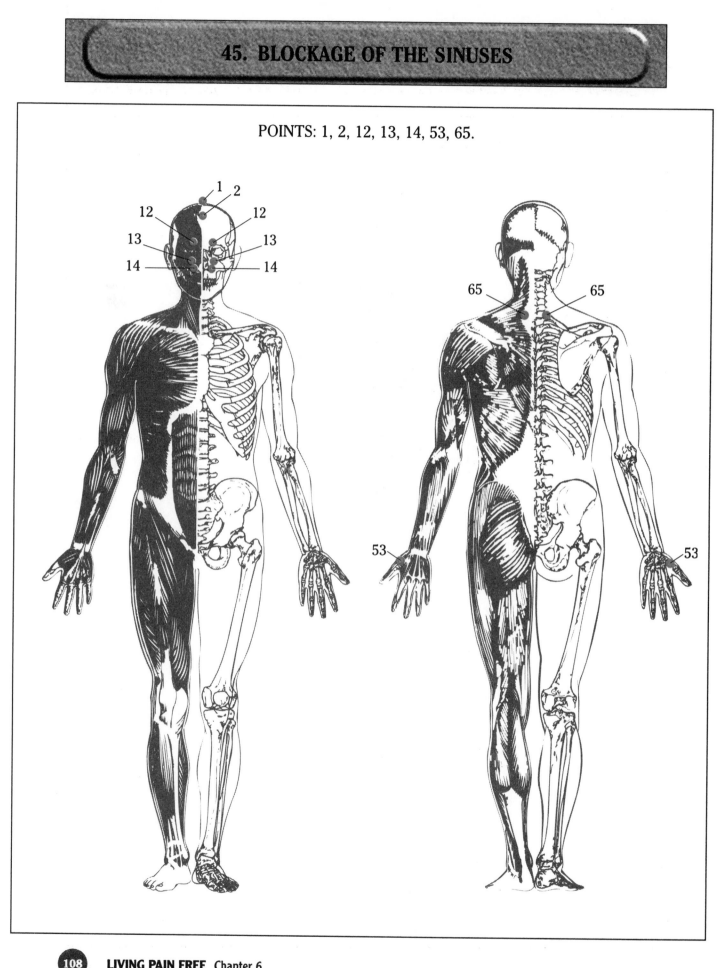

POINTS: 1, 3, 4, 12, 13, 18, 34, 35, 91, 104.

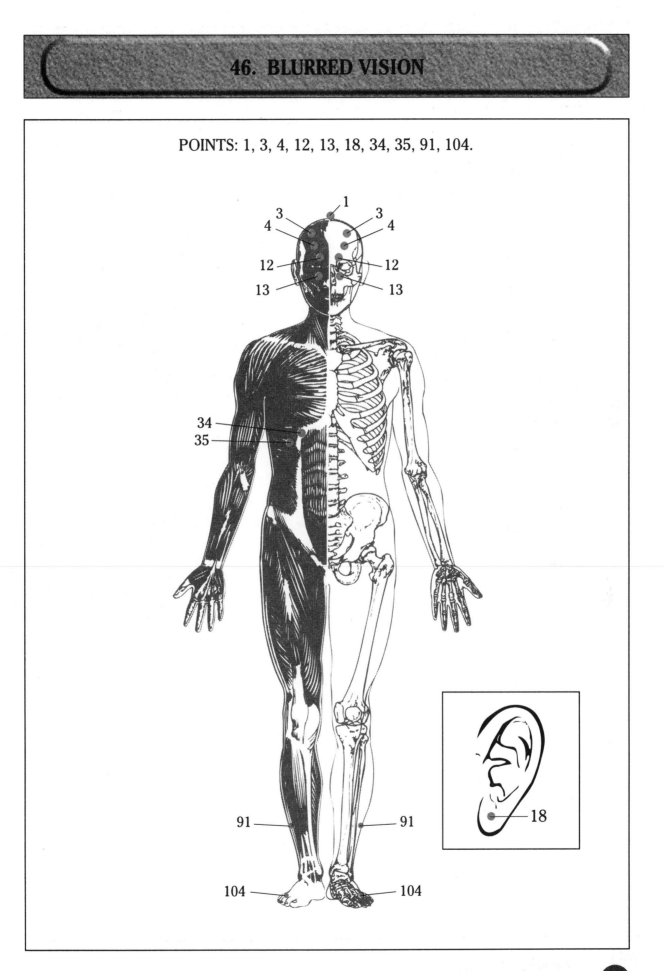

POINTS: 1, 5, 43, 48, 59, 77, 94, 98.

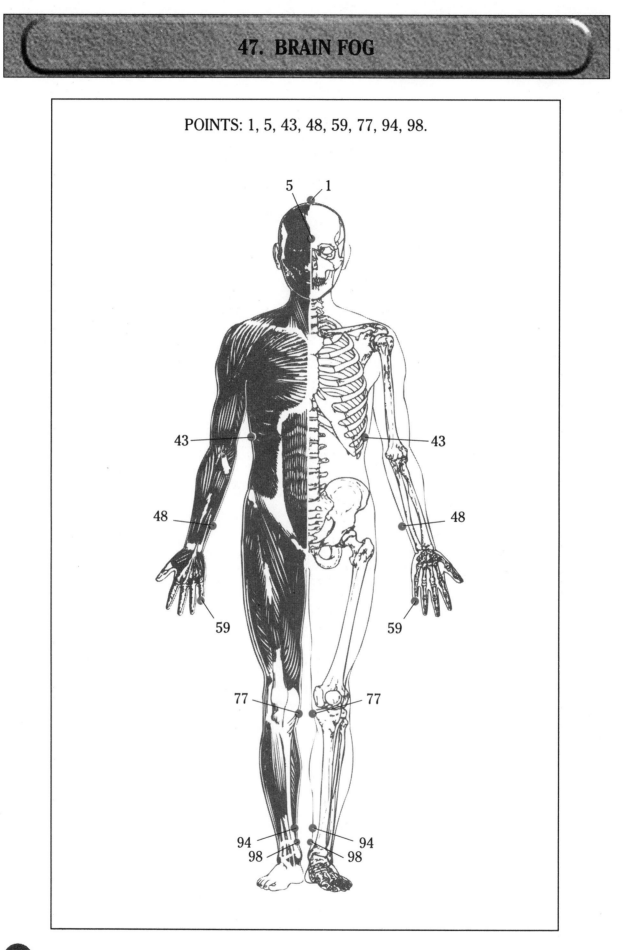

POINTS: 23, 26, 31, 46, 49, 83, 102.

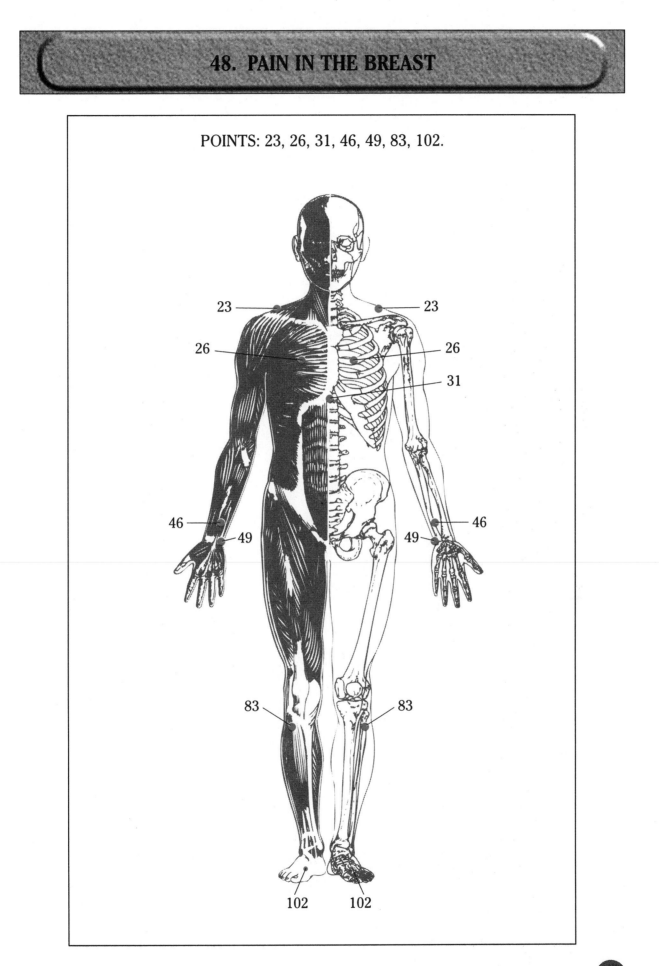

POINTS: 20, 24, 25, 45, 50, 90, 98.

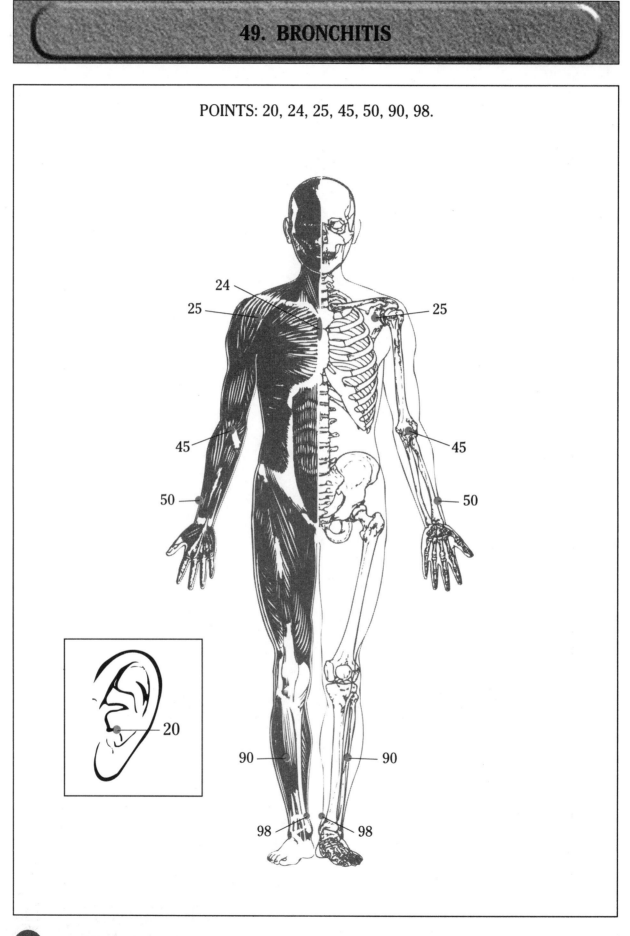

50. BULIMIA

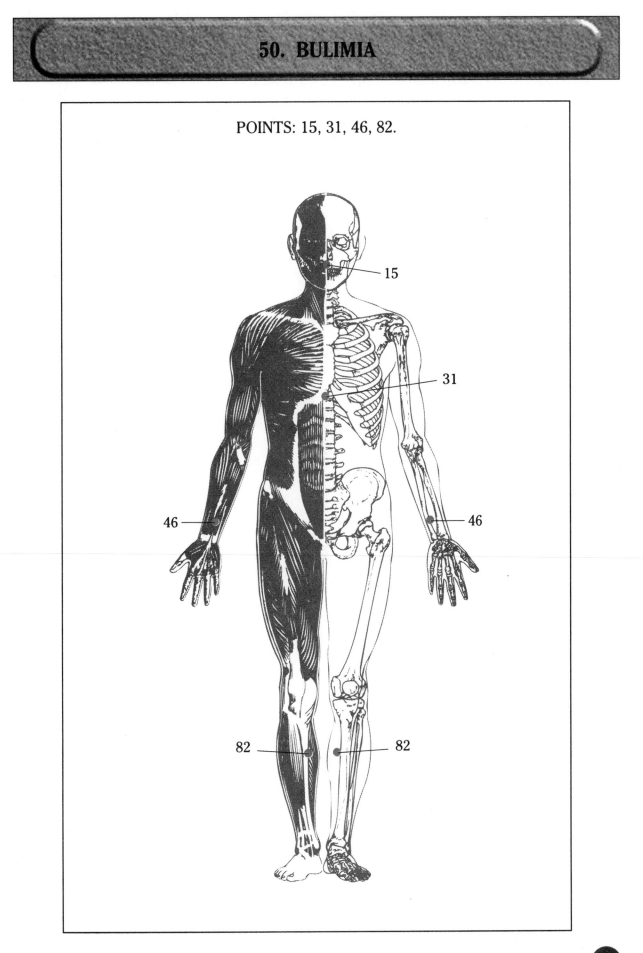

POINTS: 15, 31, 46, 82.

POINTS: 15, 21, 27, 46.

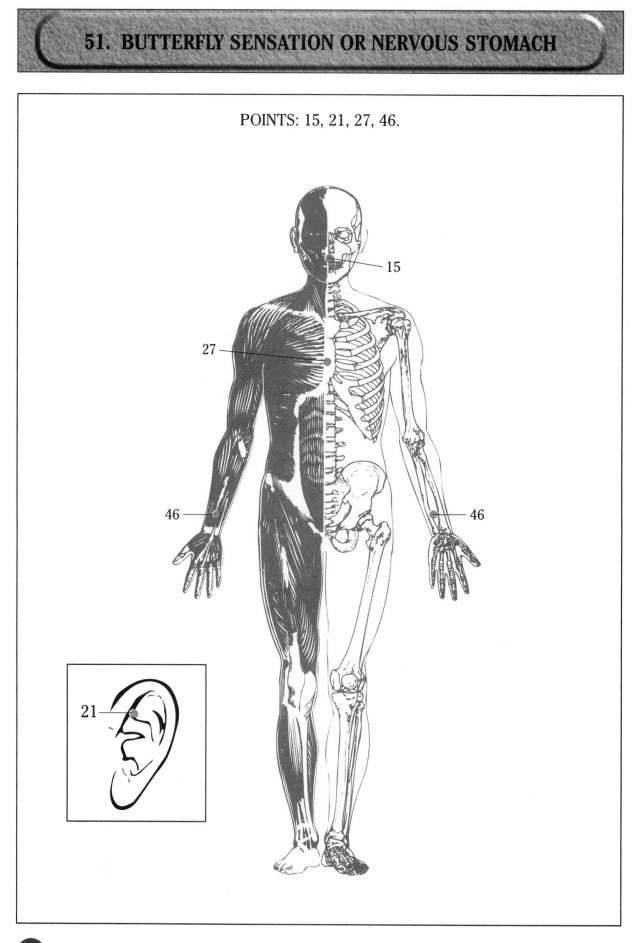

52. CARDIAC ARREST AND RESPIRATORY ARREST

POINTS: 15, 56, 58, 59, 61, 69, 70, 111.

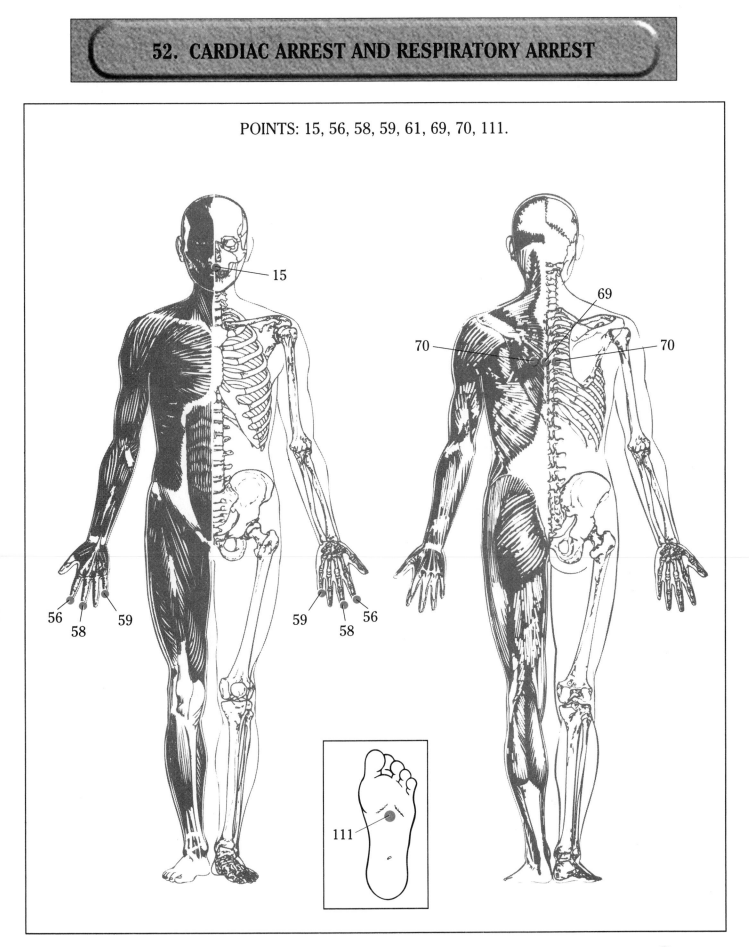

POINTS: 15, 27, 28, 46, 49, 58, 59, 69.

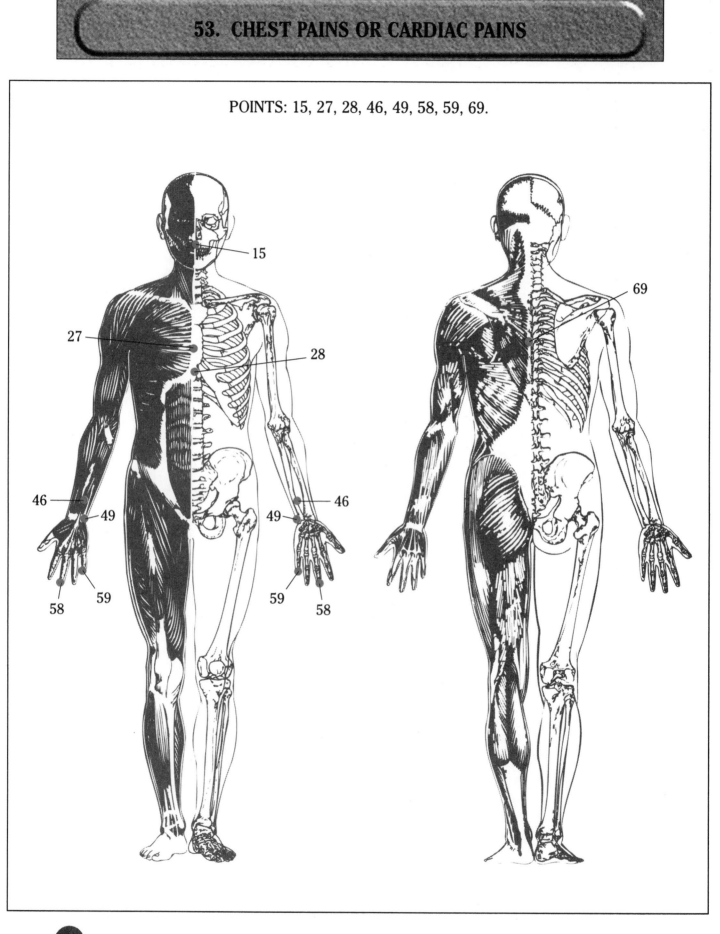

54. CELIAC SPRUE

POINTS: 36, 38, 41, 42, 87, 98, 101.

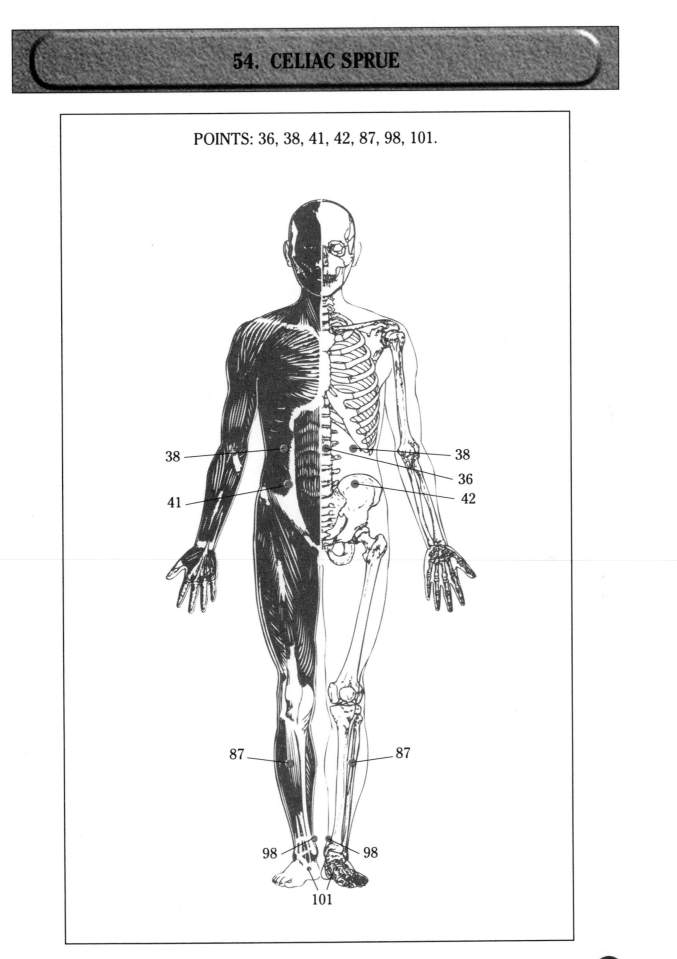

55. CHEMICAL SENSITIVITY

POINTS: 1, 24, 34, 93, 95, 96, 102.

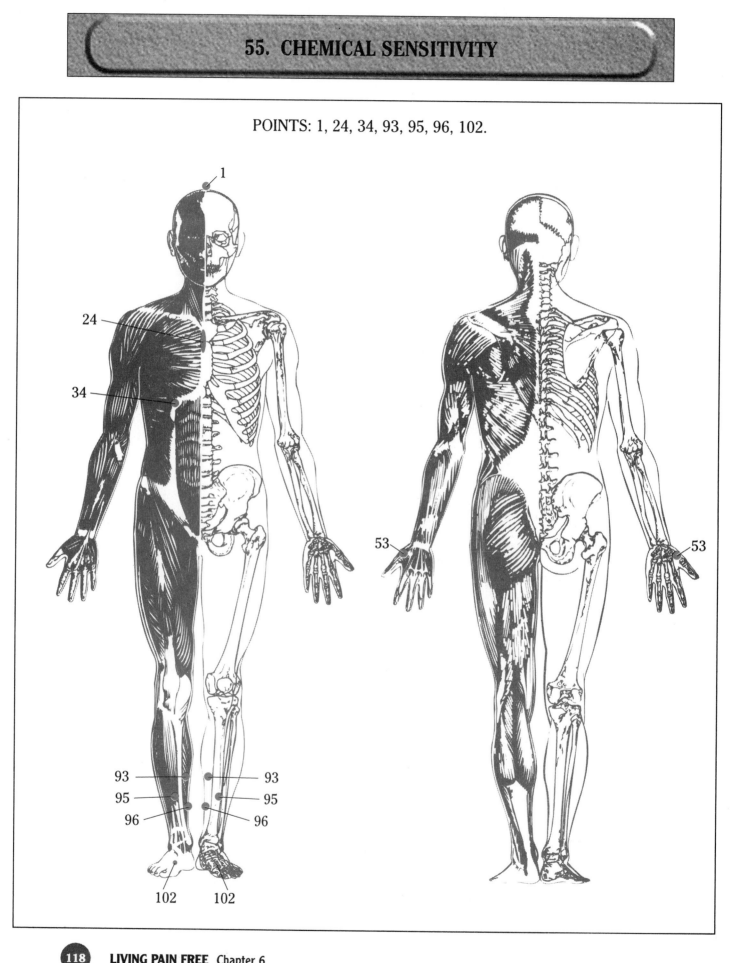

56. LUNG CONGESTION

POINTS: 25, 45, 50, 81, 90.

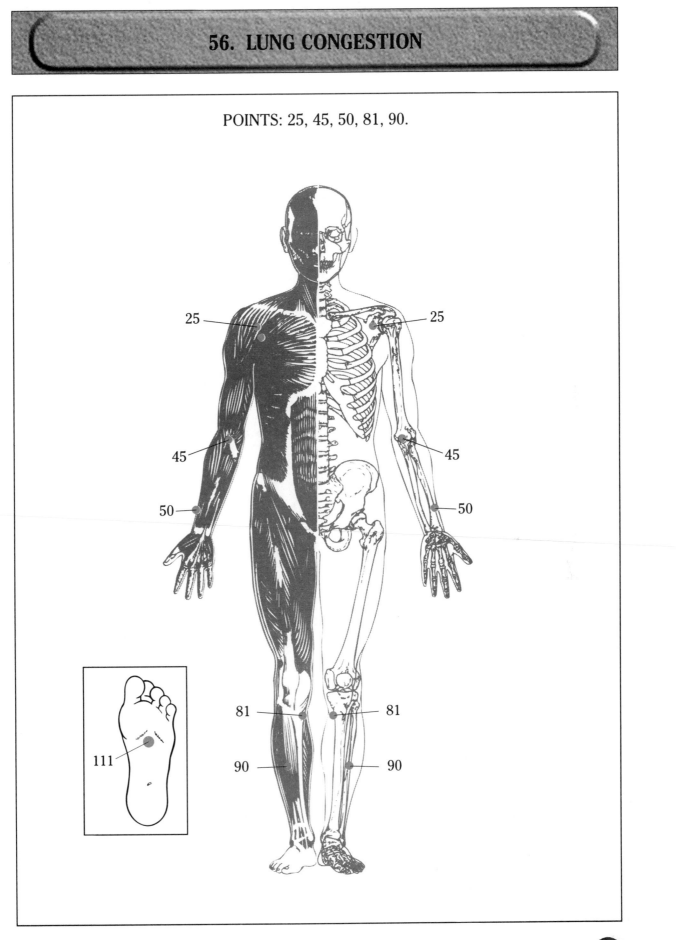

POINTS: 27, 31, 46, 49.

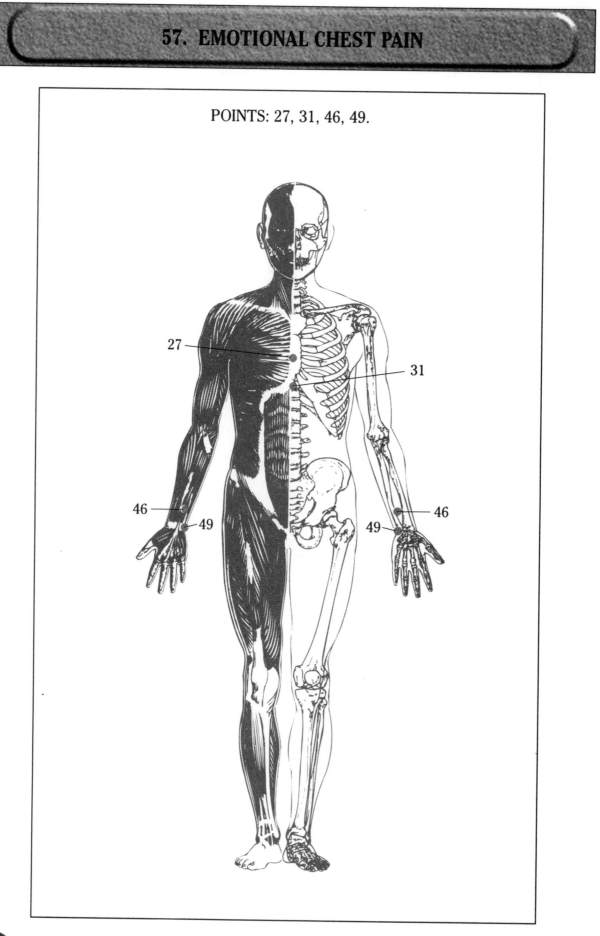

58. CONSTIPATION

POINTS: 38, 42, 83, 87.

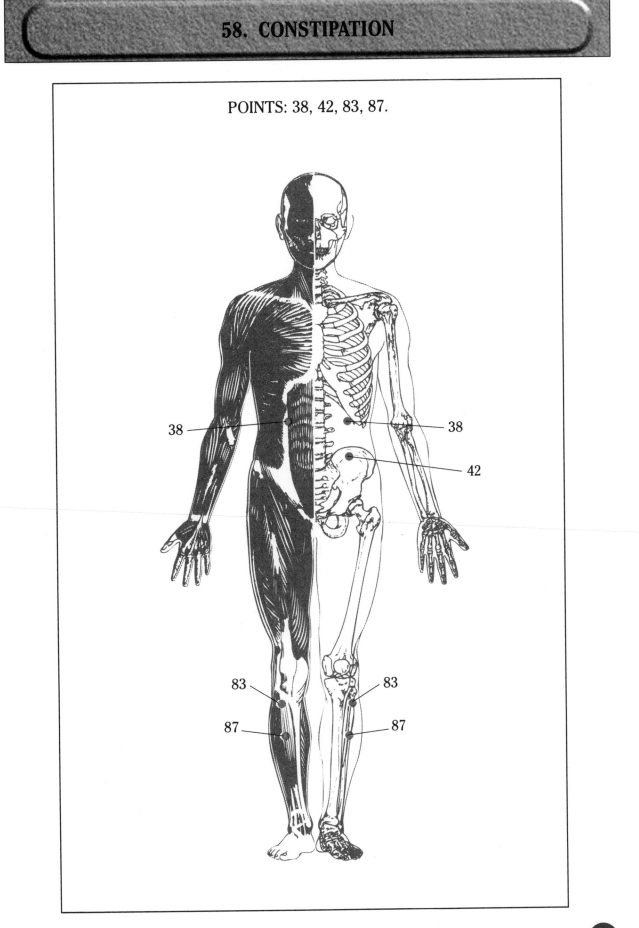

POINTS: 83, 84, 96, 98, 108.

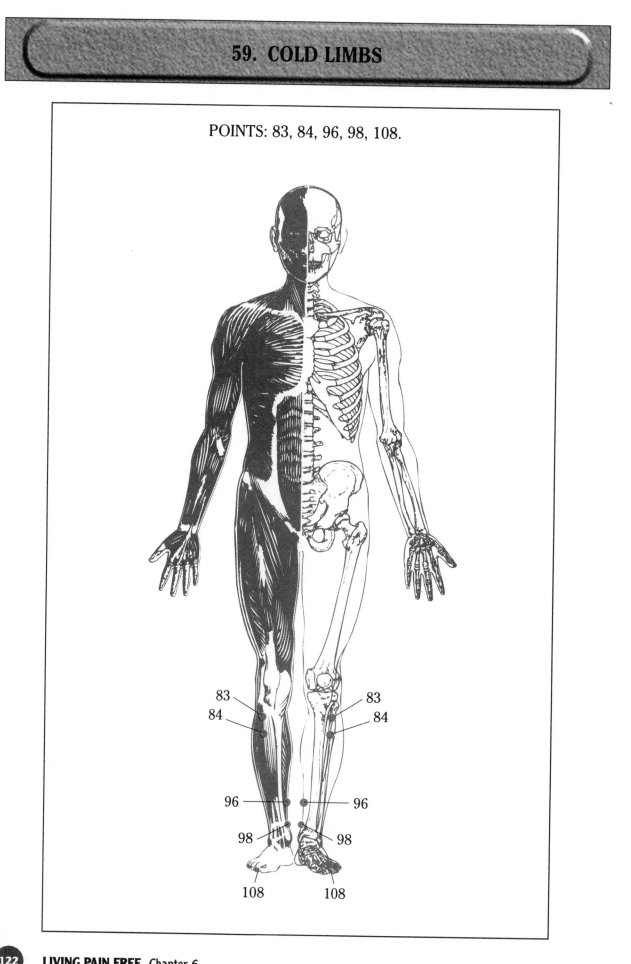

POINTS: 21, 27, 43, 46, 48, 49, 52.

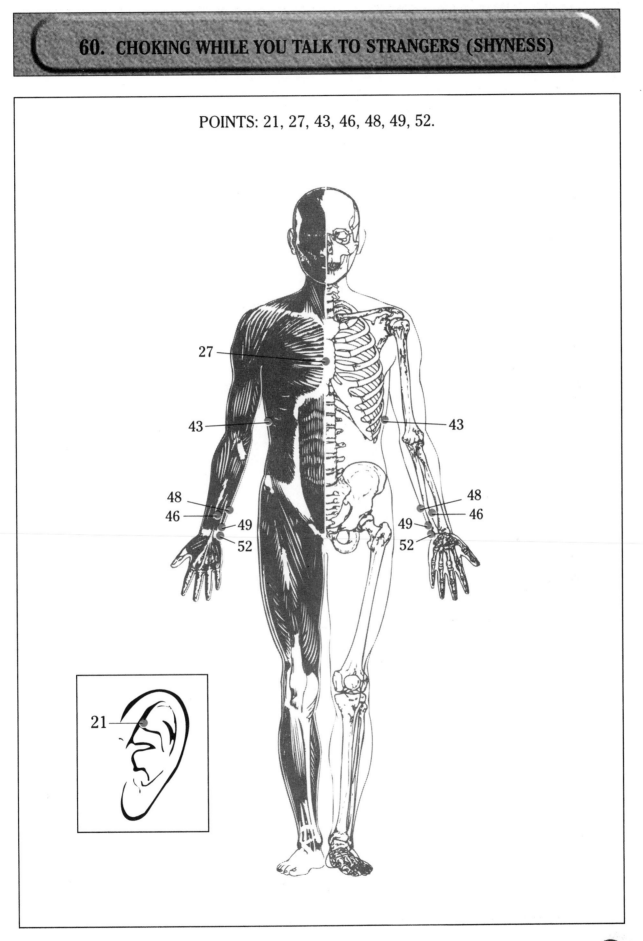

POINTS: 24, 40, 44, 66, 75, 77, 83, 94, 95, 98, 102.

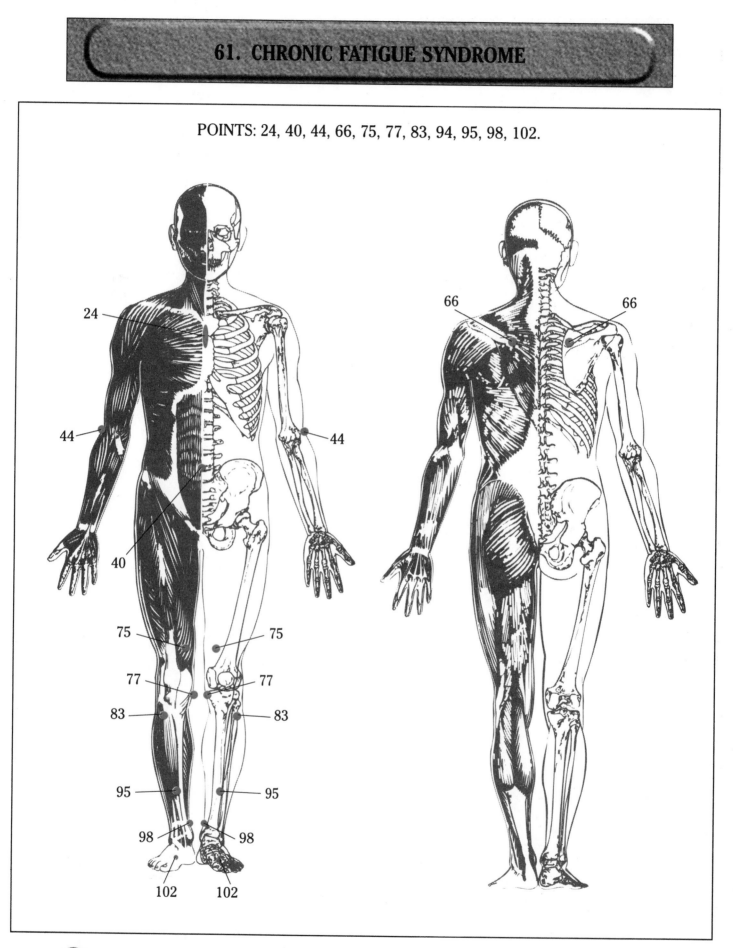

62. COMA OR SEMI-CONSCIOUSNESS

POINTS: 1, 15, 56, 58, 59, 61, 63, 111.

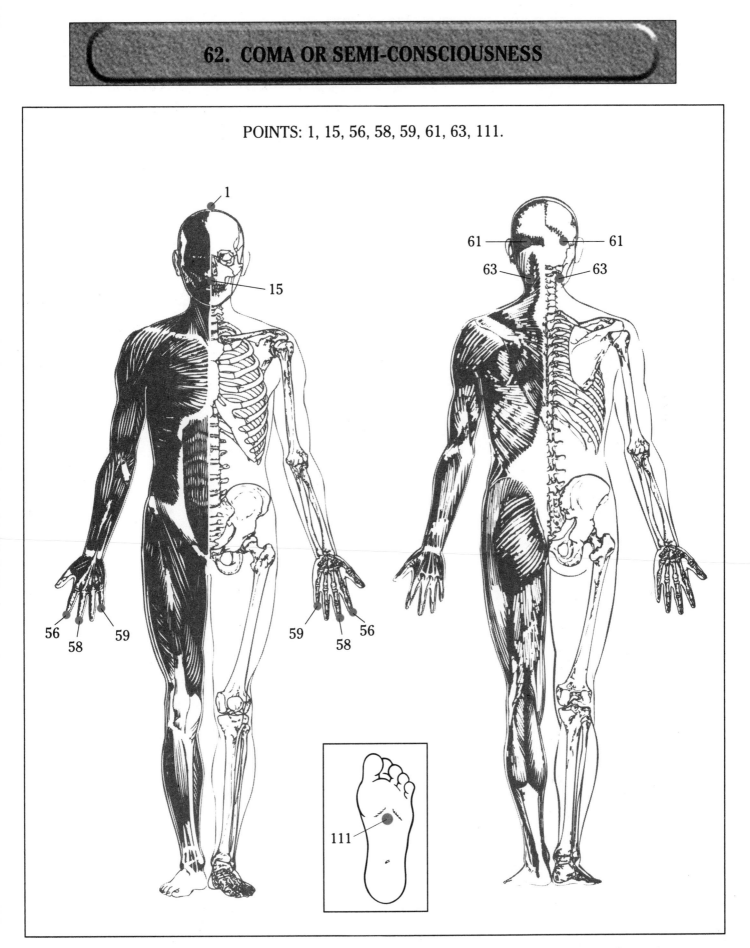

POINTS: 38, 57, 87, 101.

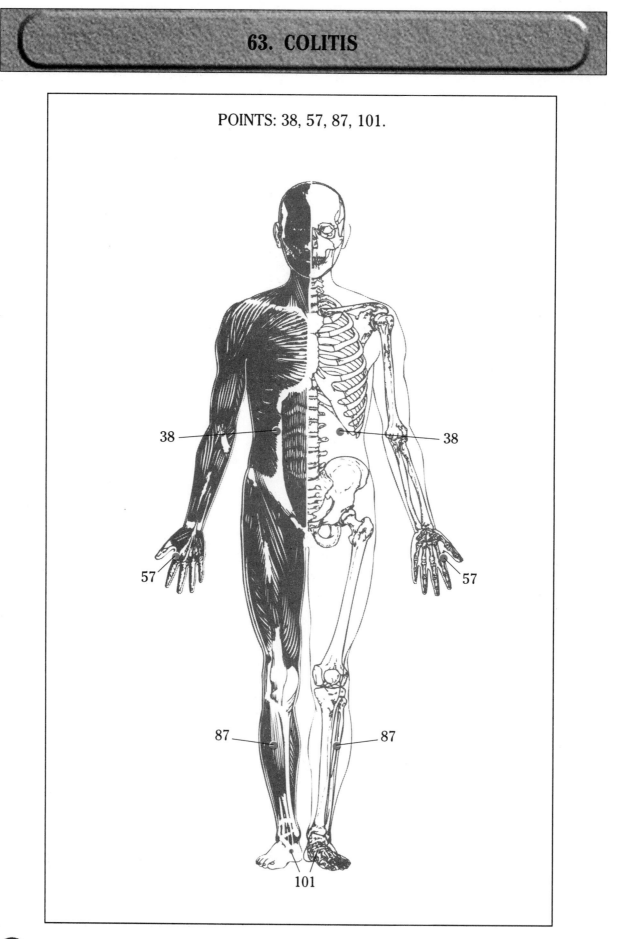

POINTS: 31, 44, 57, 75, 88.

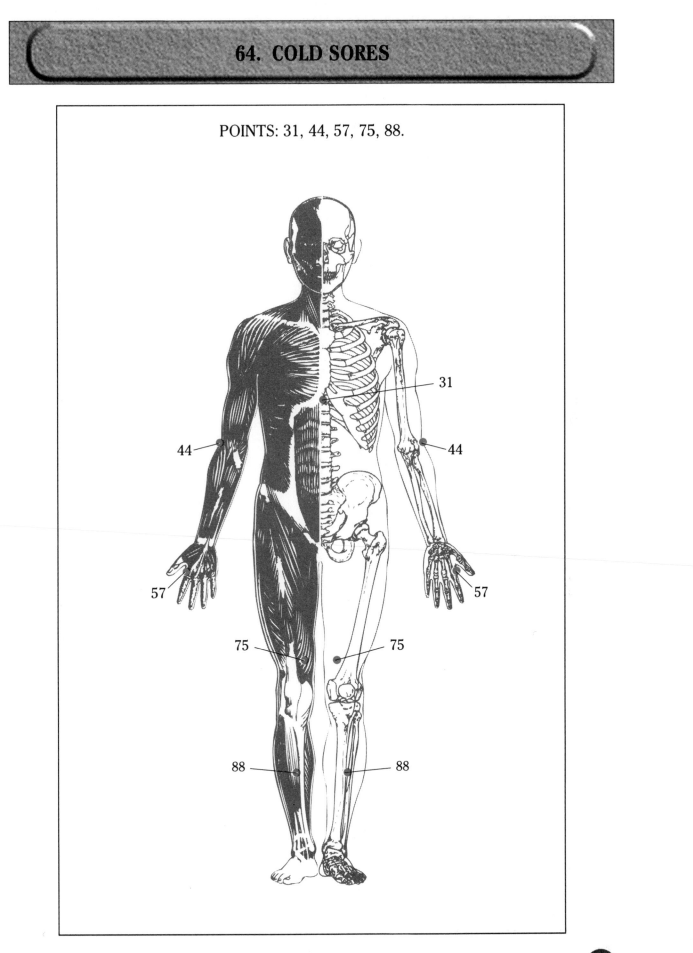

POINTS: 1, 2, 3, 4, 14, 63, 87, 97, 104.

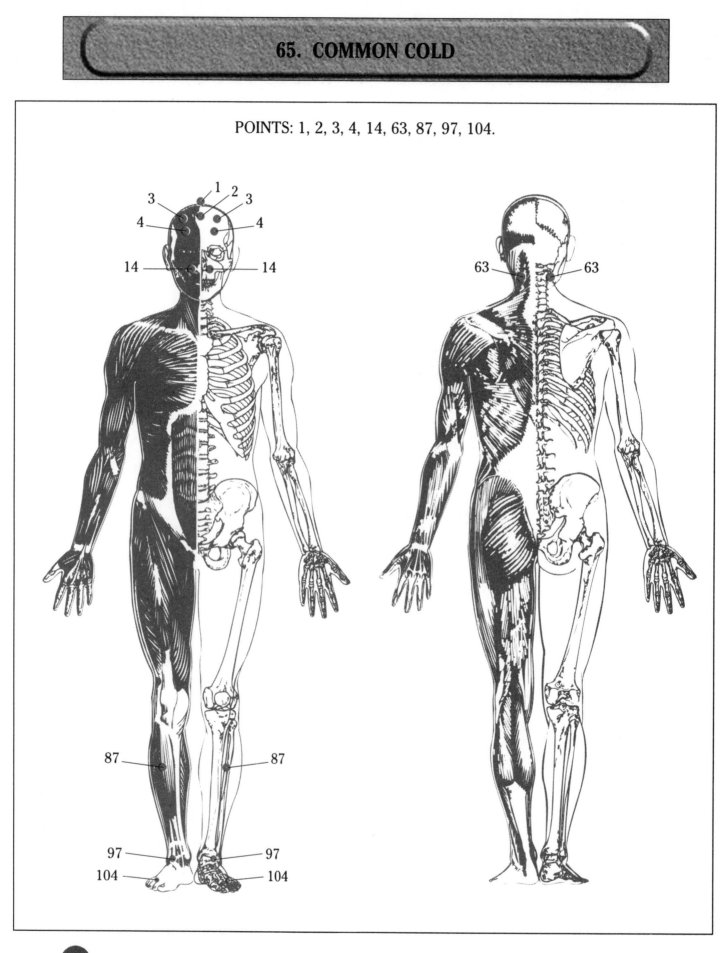

66. CONVULSIONS

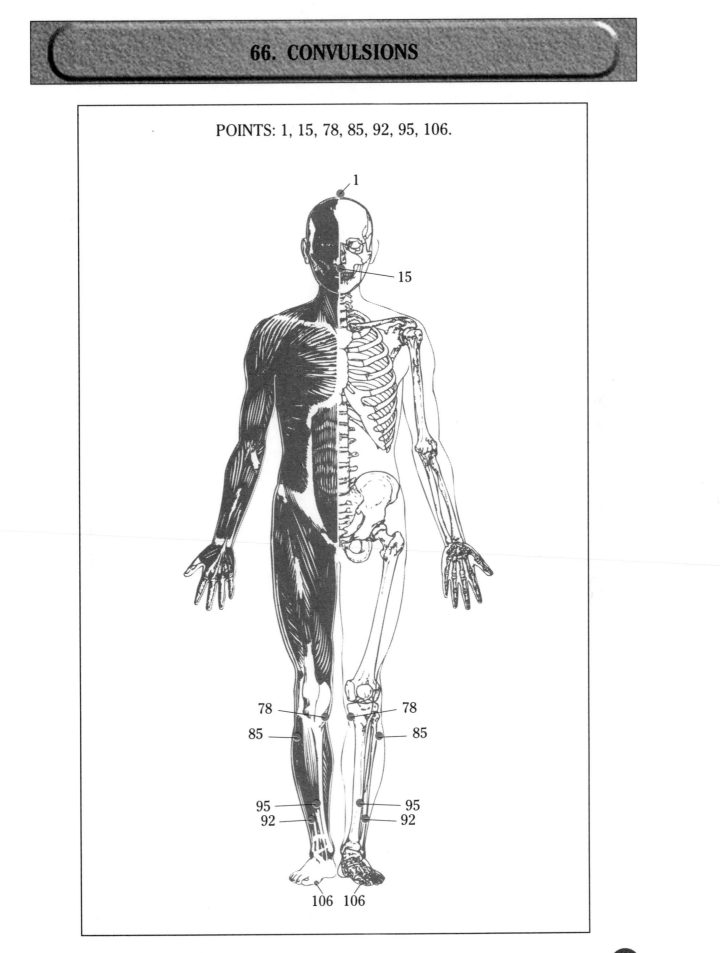

POINTS: 1, 15, 78, 85, 92, 95, 106.

POINTS: 25, 26, 50, 64, 65, 66, 69, 90.

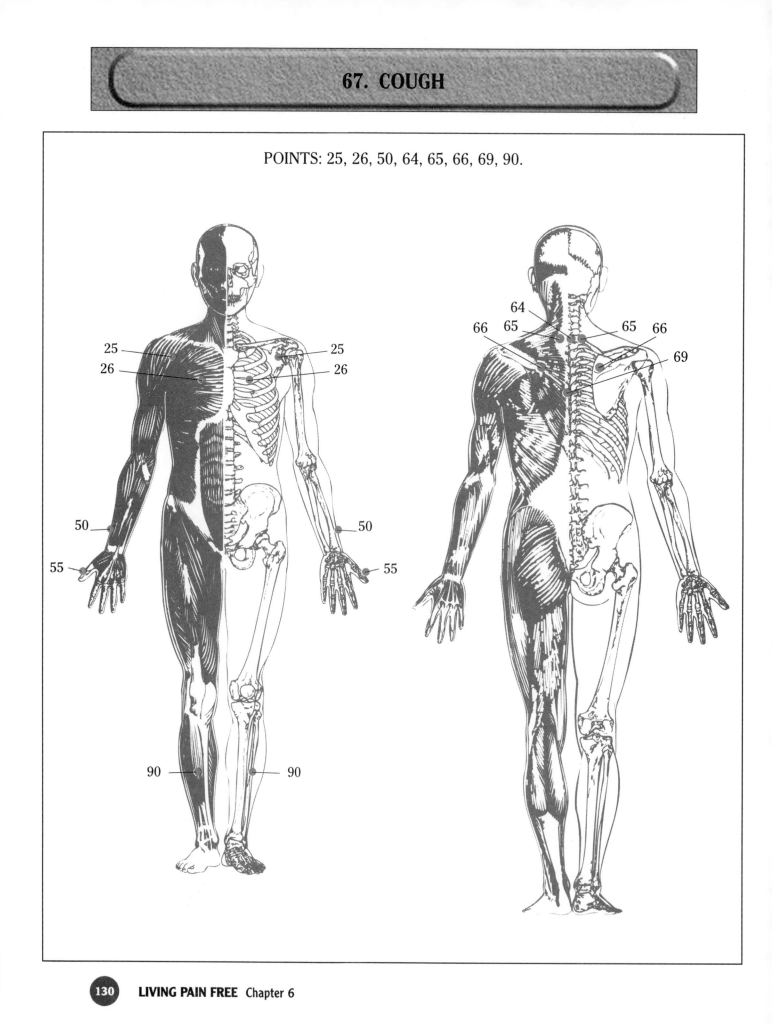

68. CRAMPS IN THE LEGS

POINTS: 79, 80, 81, 88, 92, 95, 96.

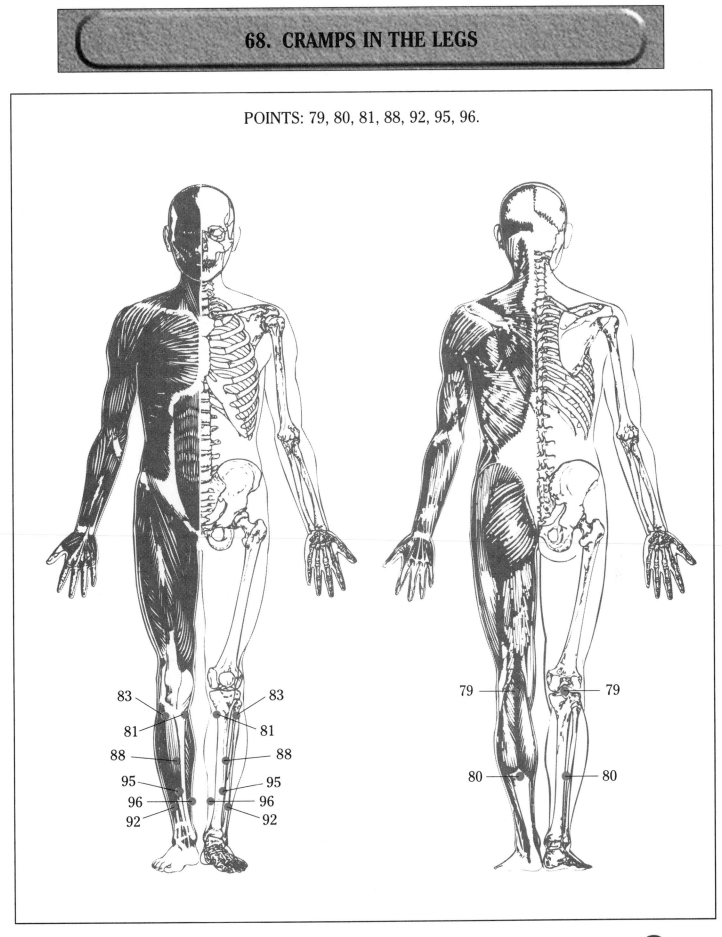

POINTS: 40, 53, 57, 87.

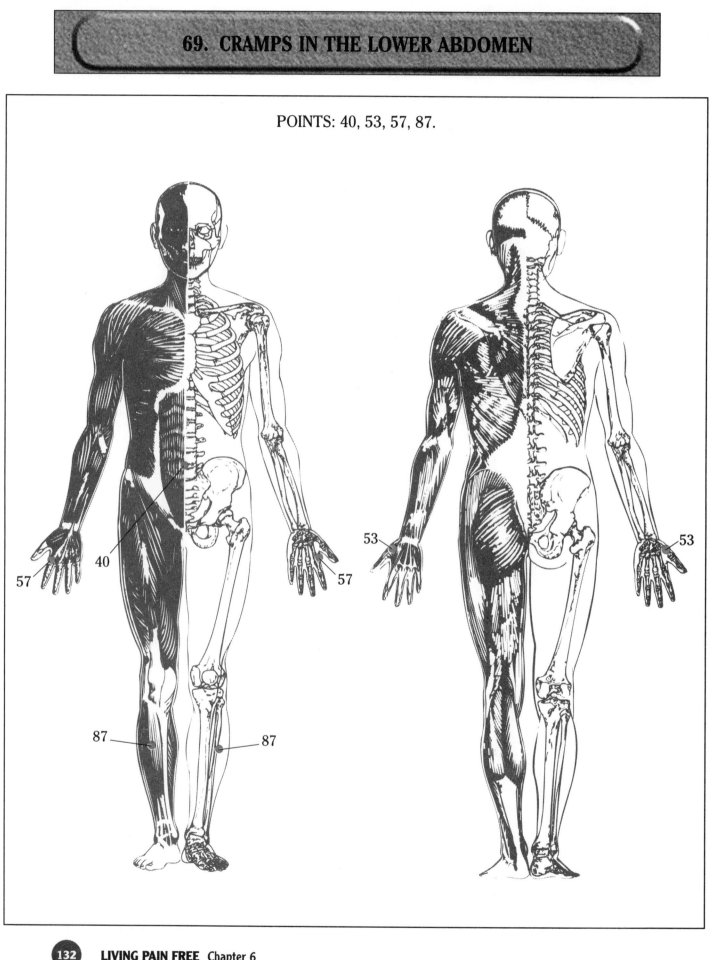

POINTS: 38, 40, 87, 88, 101.

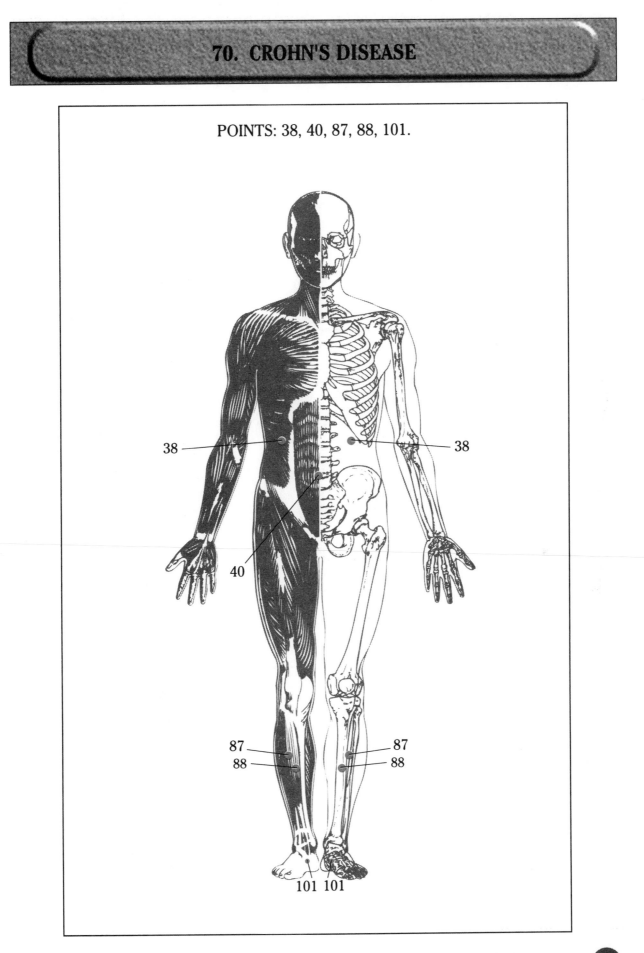

POINTS: 27, 28, 34, 46, 48, 49.

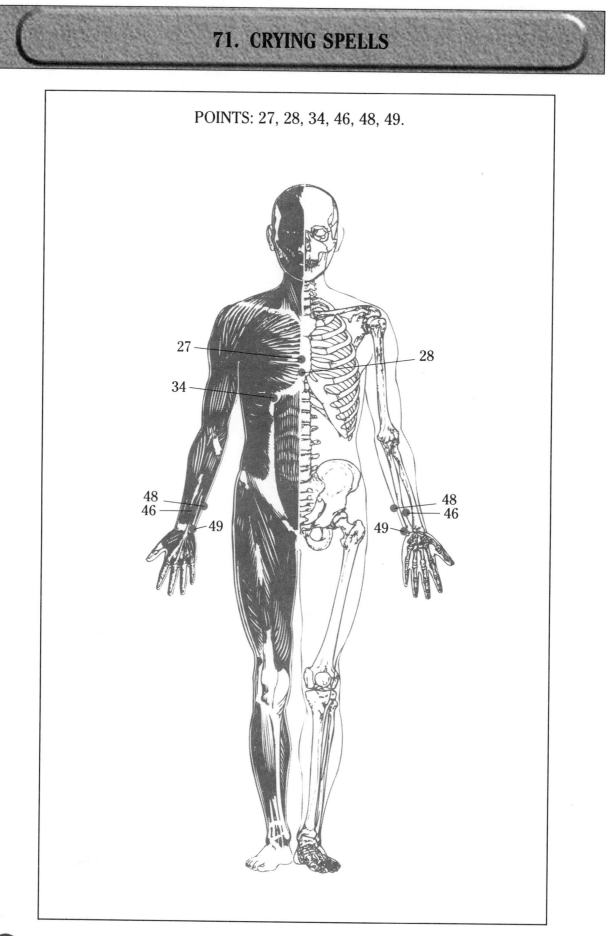

POINTS: 9, 11, 47, 54, 51, 98, 73, 96, 97.

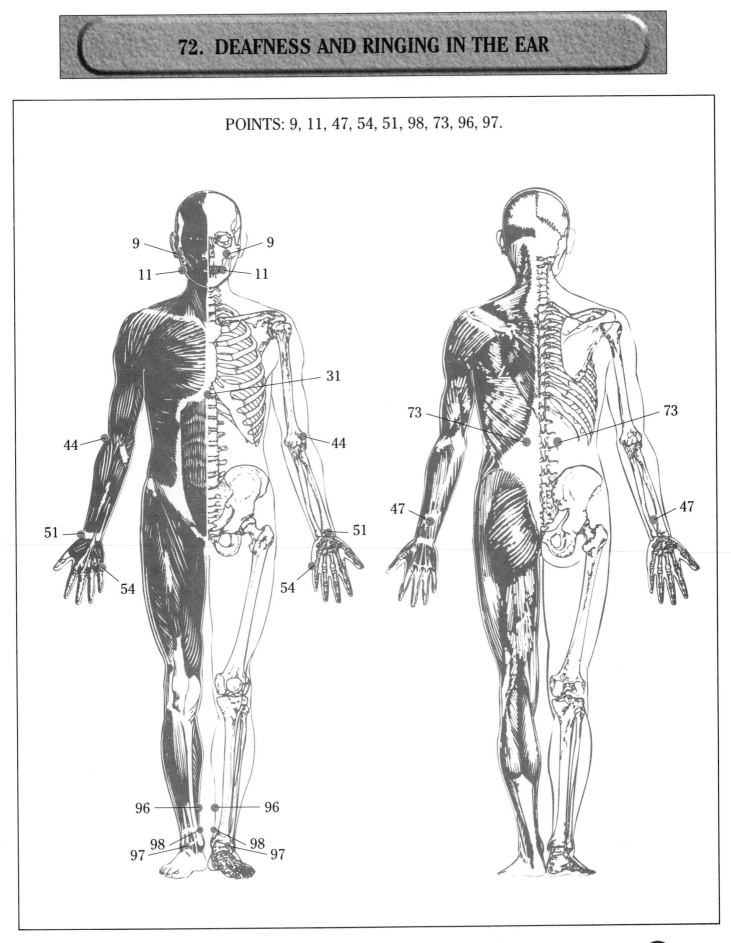

POINTS: 31, 44, 46, 49, 96, 97.

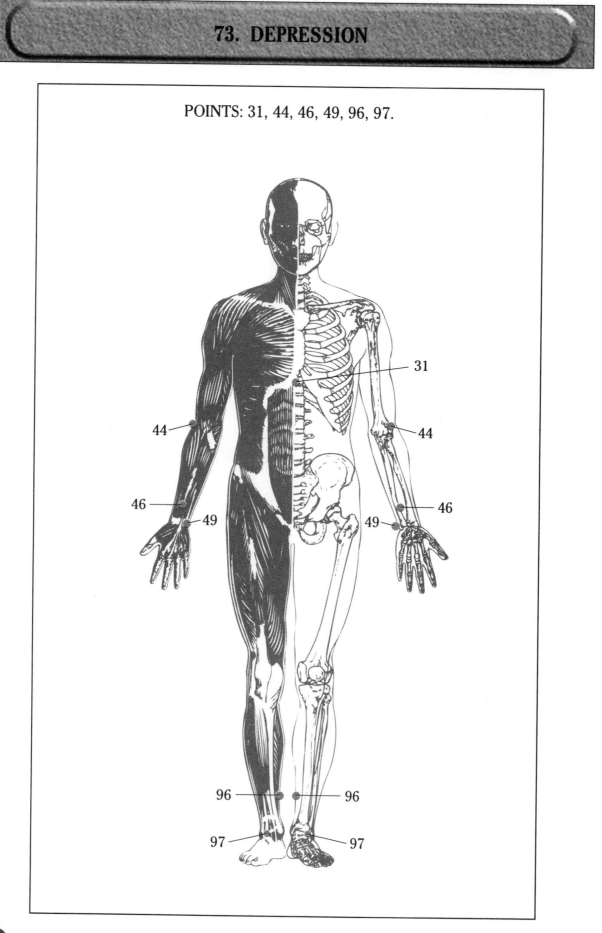

74. DIARRHEA

POINTS: 31, 36, 37, 38, 39, 40, 44, 71, 72, 82, 84, 87, 102, 106.

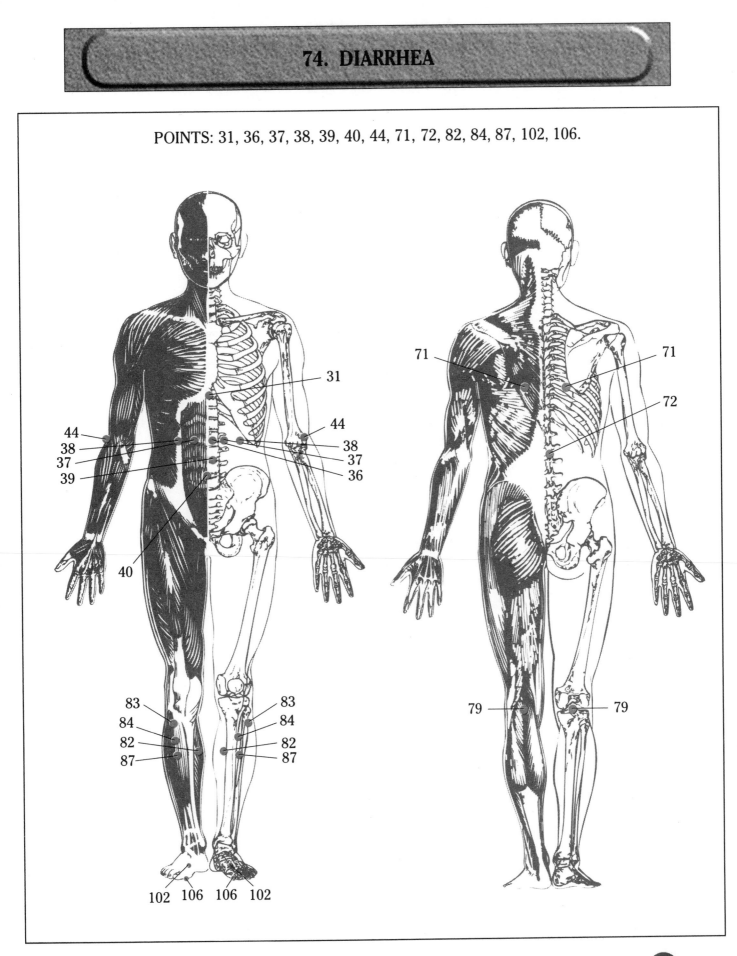

POINTS: 15, 25, 26, 28, 29, 39, 45, 50, 61, 64, 65, 66, 90, 98.

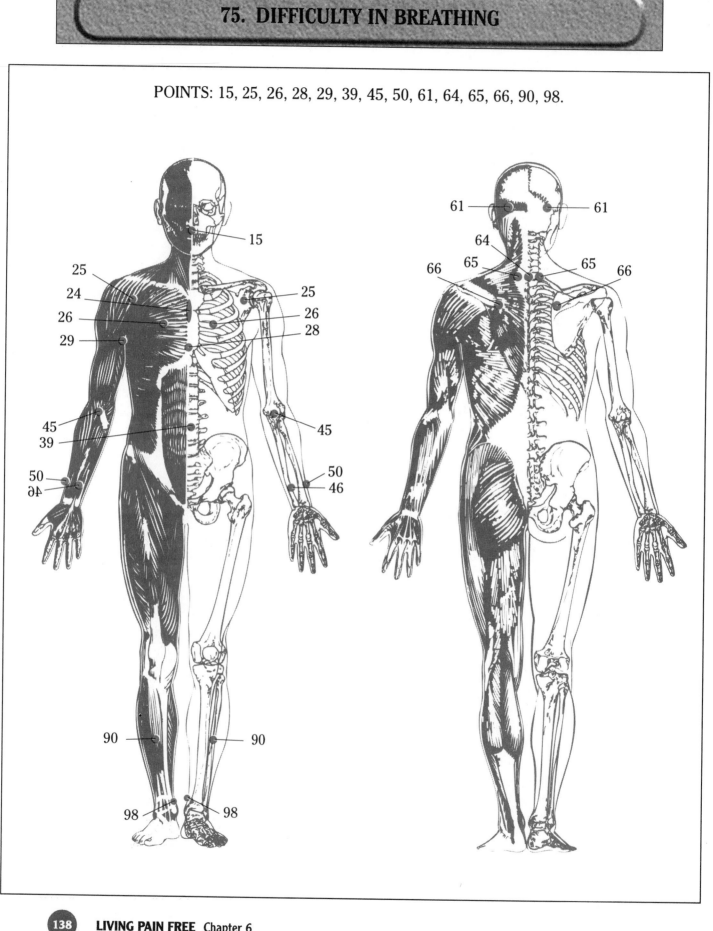

POINTS: 27, 28, 31, 34, 54, 64, 93.

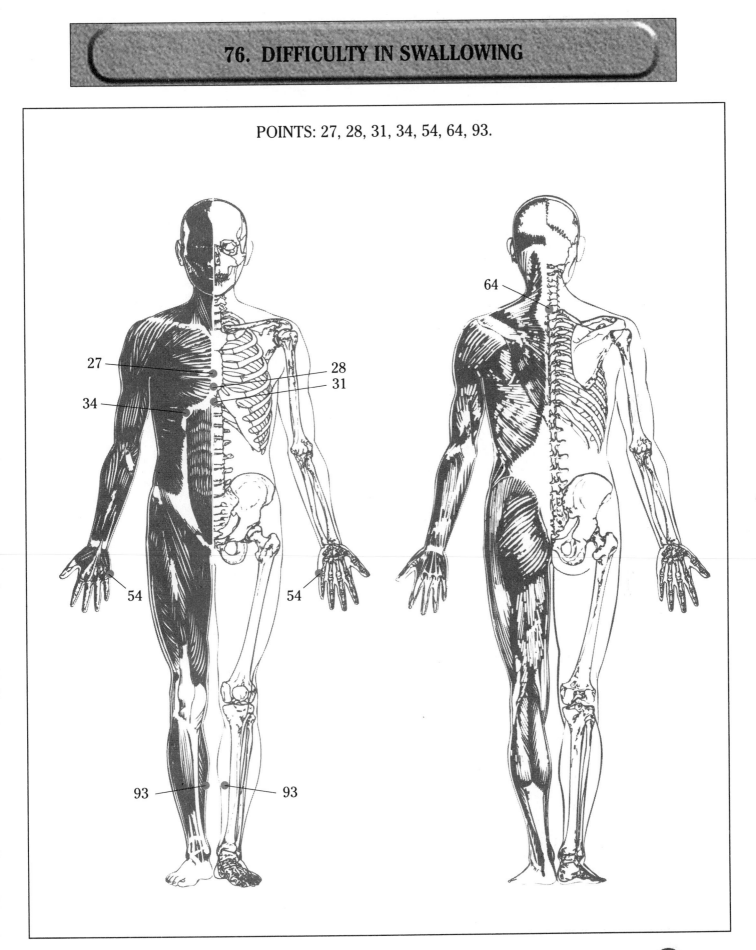

POINTS: 41, 76, 78, 81, 82, 92, 95, 107.

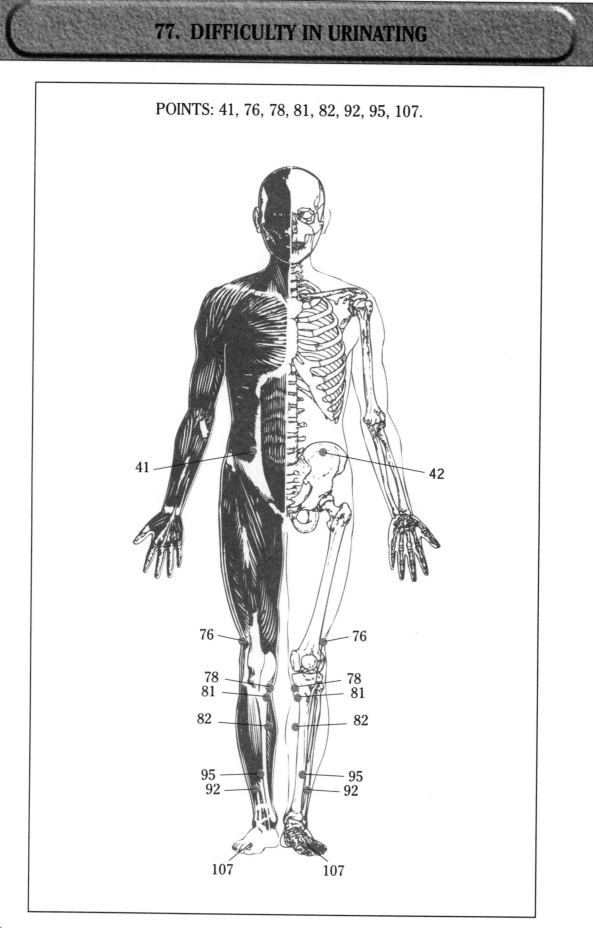

POINTS: 4, 5, 7, 9, 13.

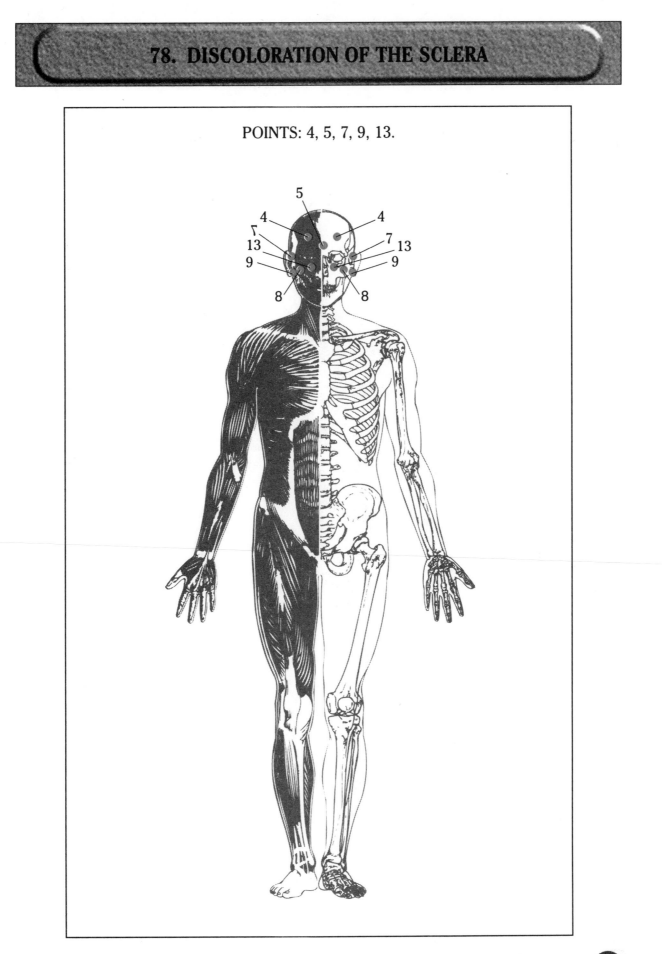

POINTS: 1, 38, 42, 87, 101.

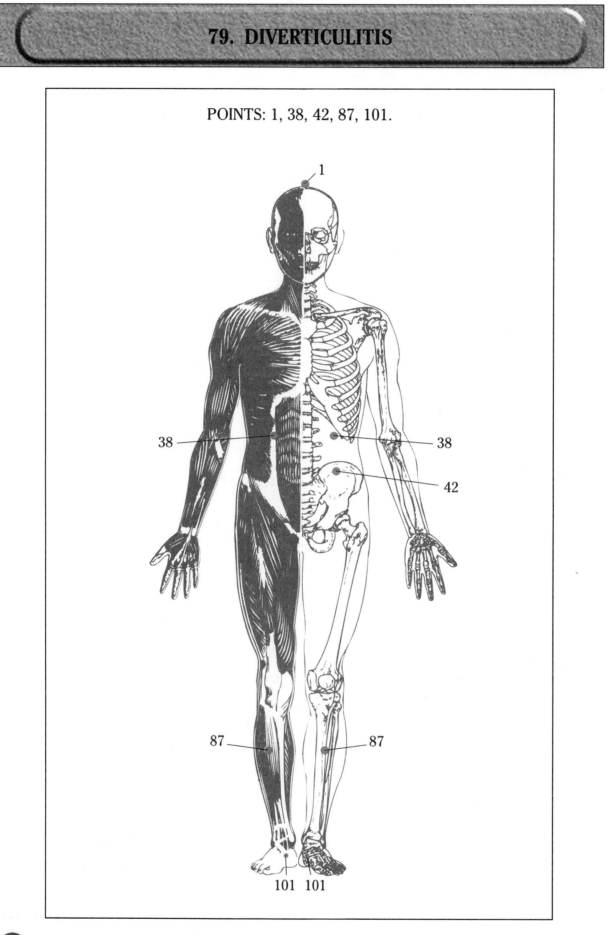

80. DIZZINESS

POINTS: 15, 24, 40, 44, 66, 75, 77, 83, 94, 95, 98, 102.

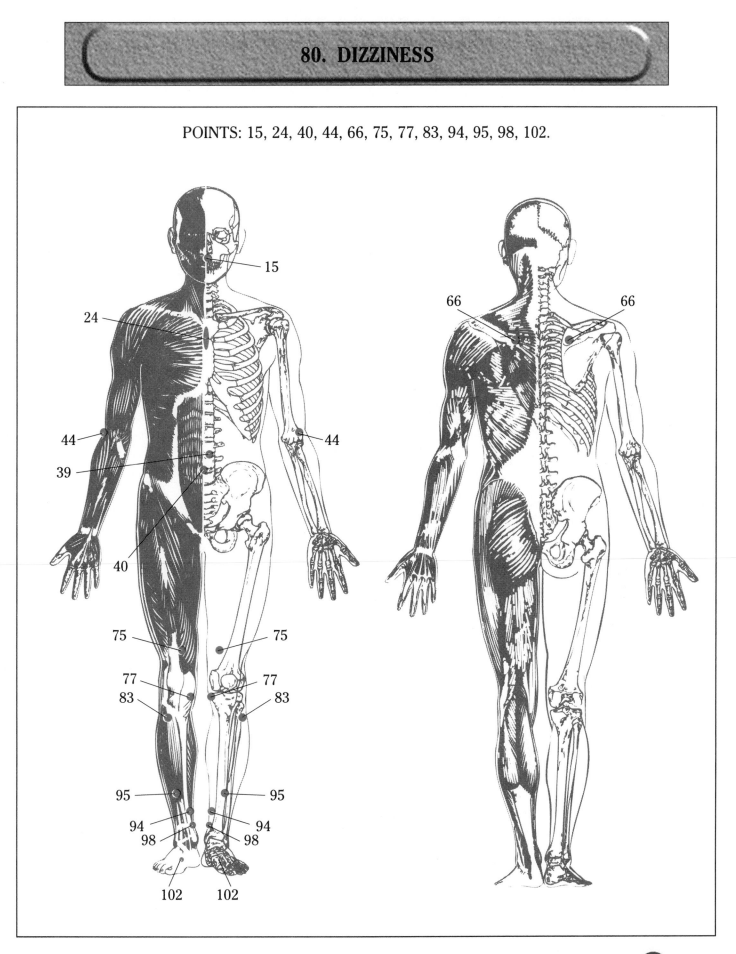

POINTS: 87, 106, 108, 109.

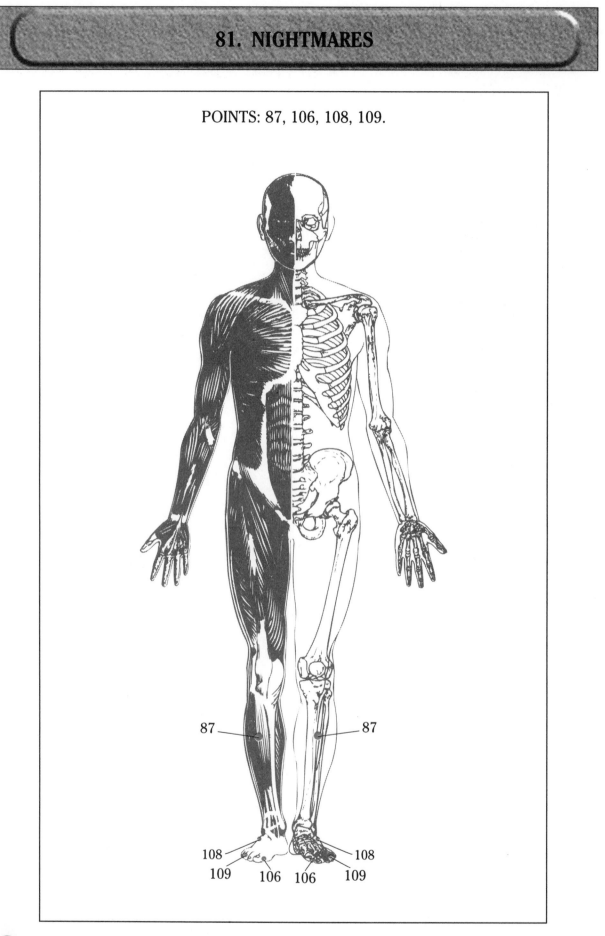

POINTS: 15, 17, 24, 31, 39, 49, 75, 96.

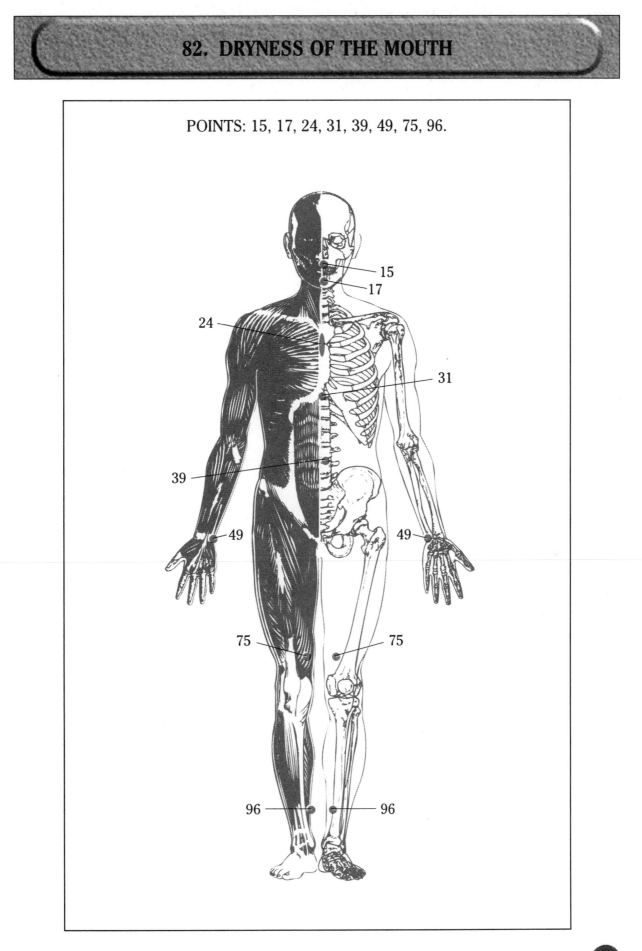

POINTS: 1, 14, 15, 17, 21, 111.

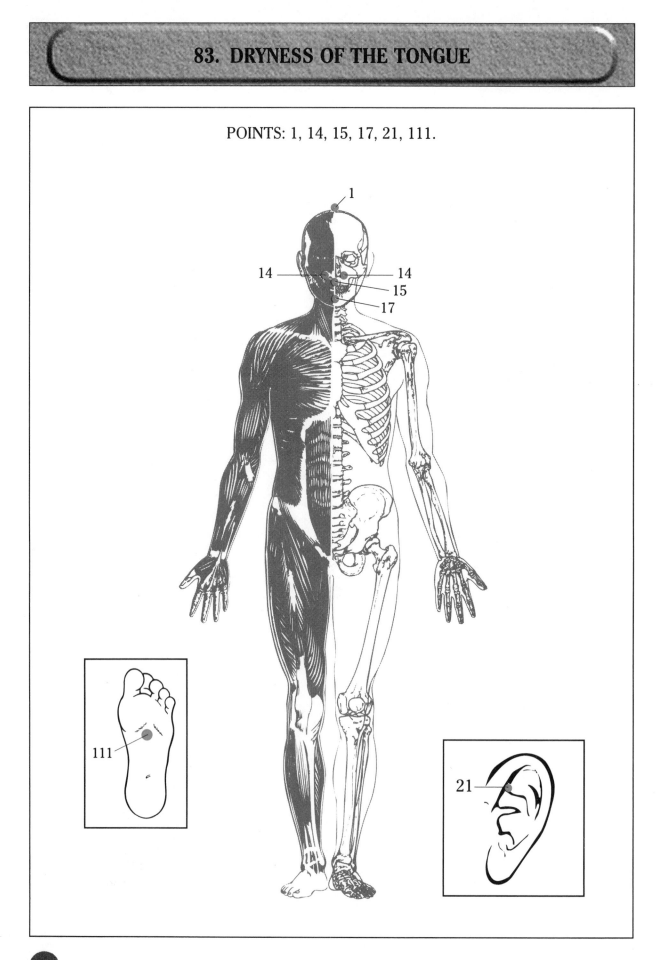

POINTS: 31, 44, 71, 82, 87, 88, 106.

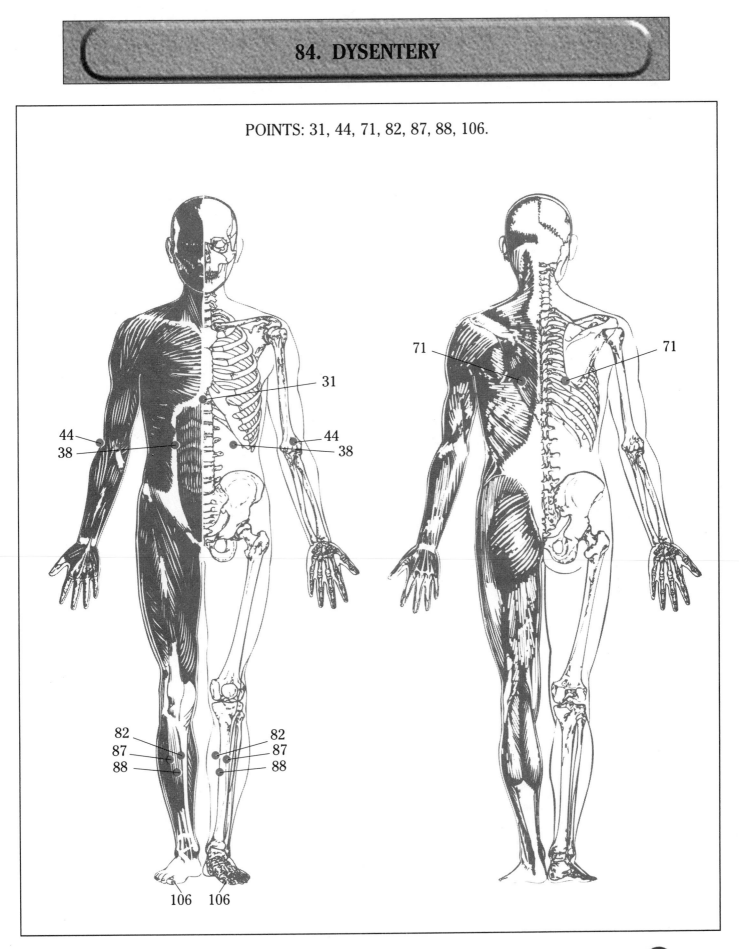

POINTS: 40, 46, 53, 77, 96, 102.

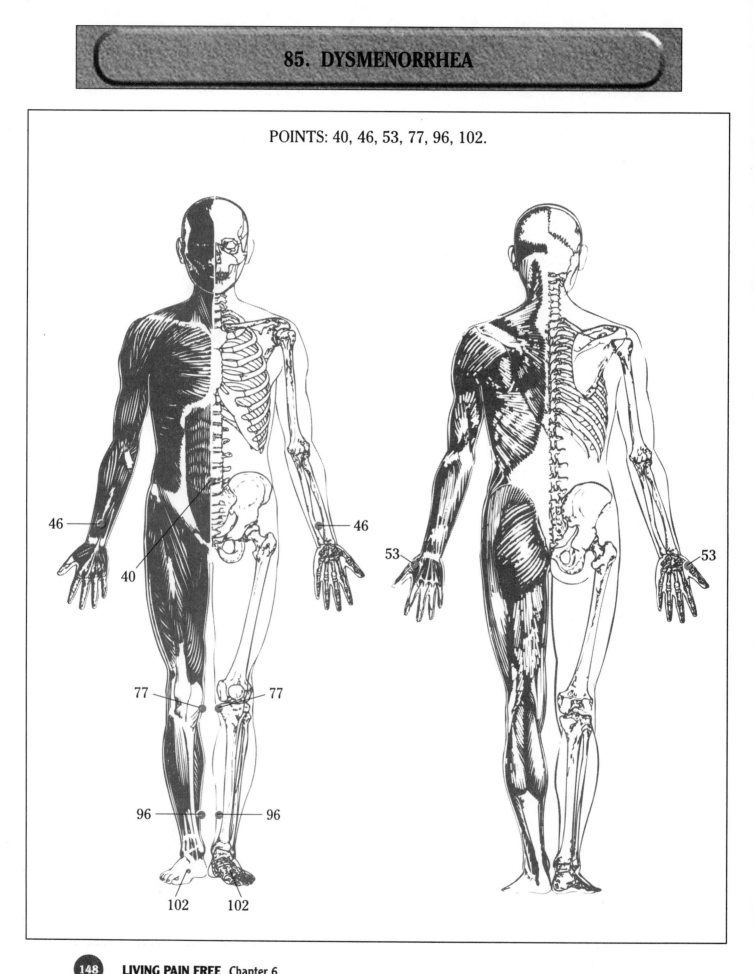

86. EARACHE

POINTS: 8, 11, 44, 47, 93.

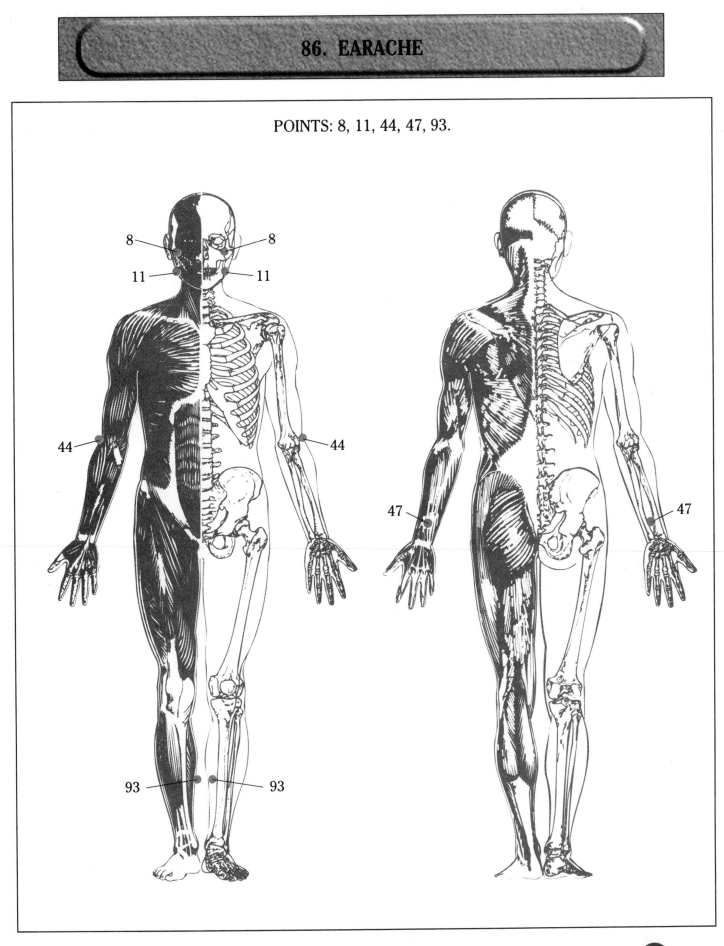

POINTS: 8, 11, 44, 46, 47, 93.

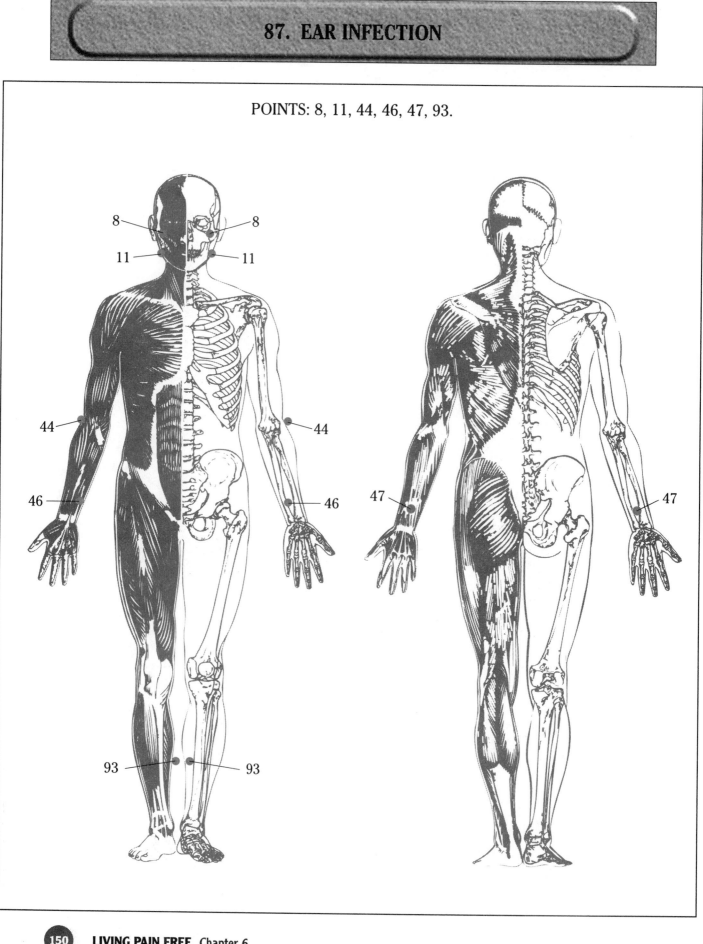

88. EATING DISORDERS

POINTS: 31, 44, 46, 53, 83, 96, 102.

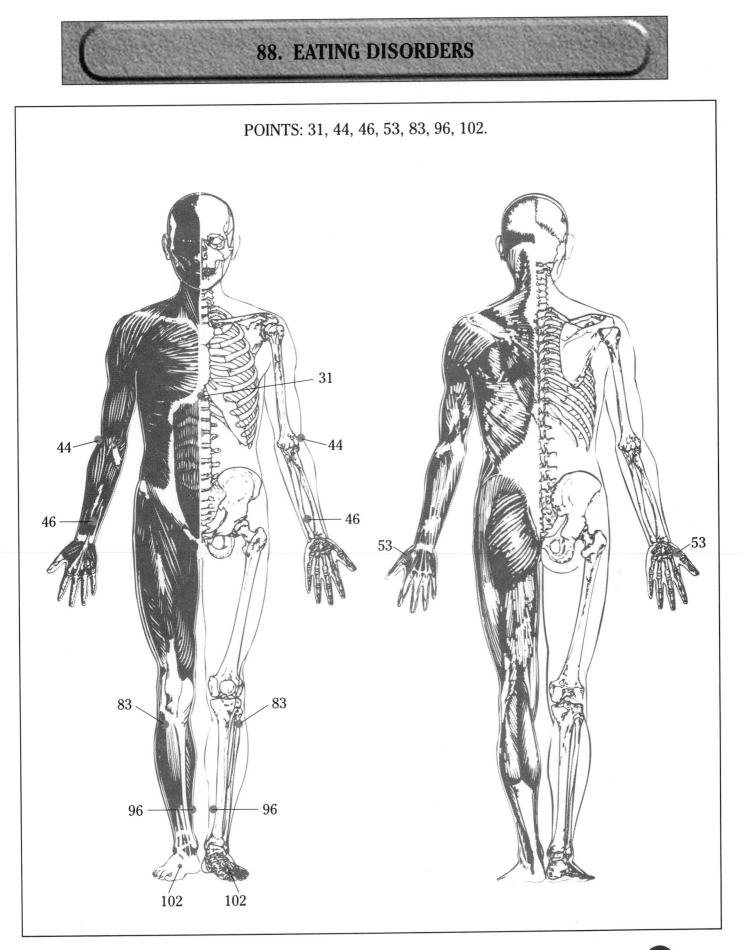

89. ECZEMA

POINTS: 10, 44, 46, 75, 78, 79.

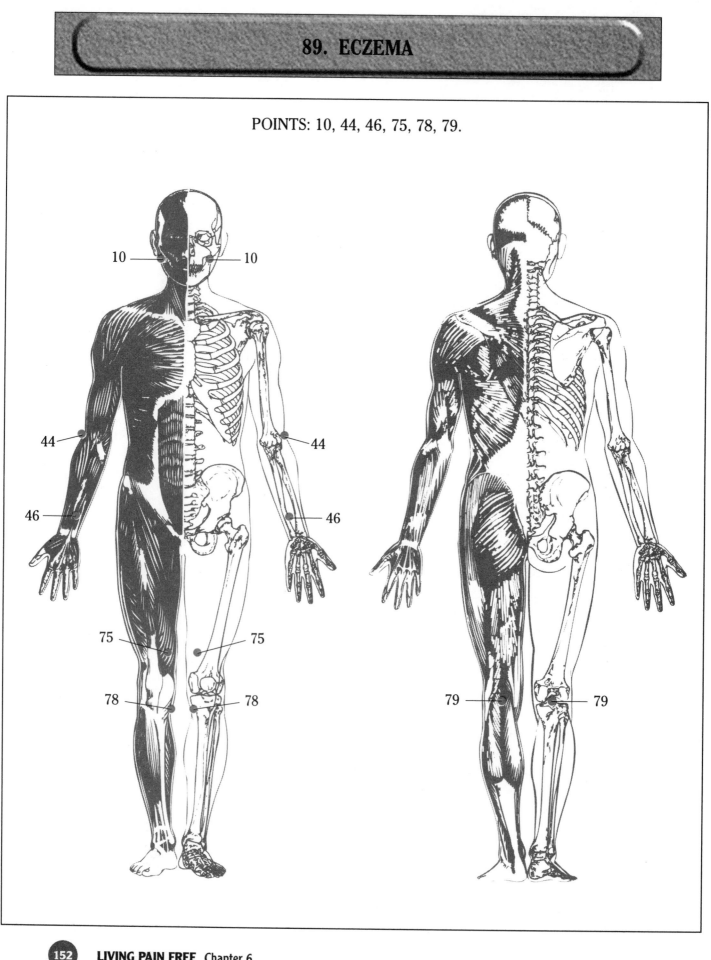

90. EDEMA

POINTS: 39, 80, 81, 82, 88, 90.

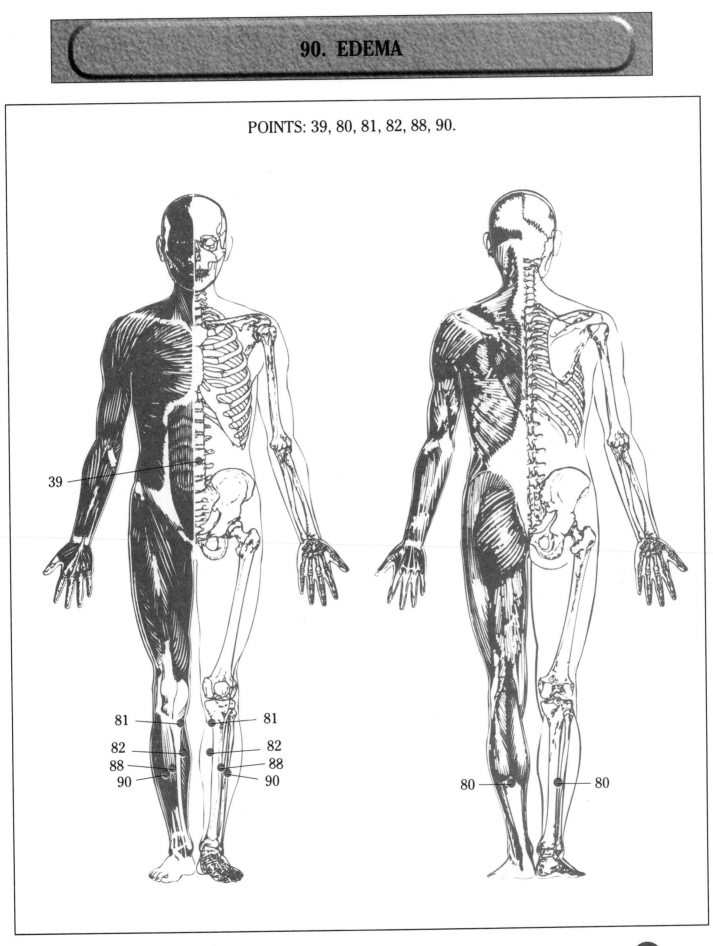

POINTS: 1, 4, 5, 15, 44, 46, 69, 102.

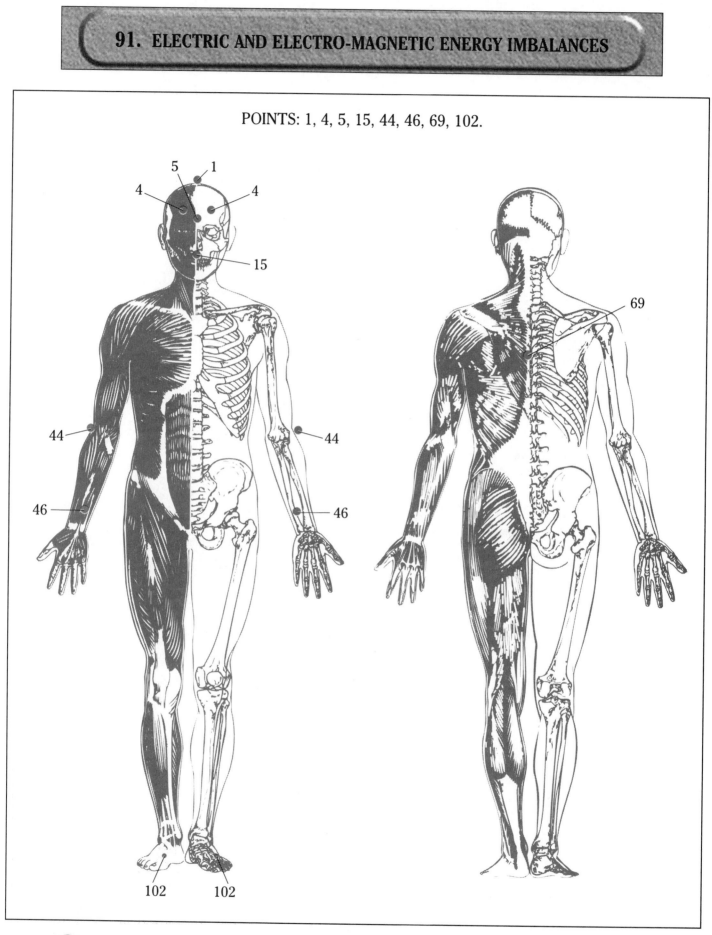

POINTS: 1, 14, 15, 25, 63, 66, 95, 102.

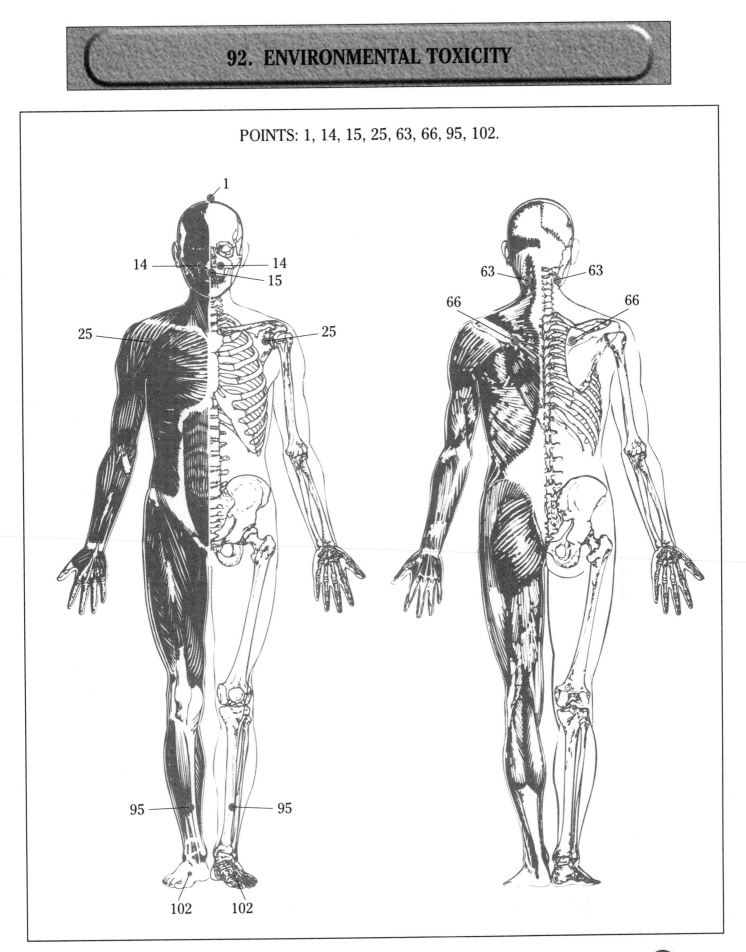

POINTS: 12, 13, 18, 91, 92, 109.

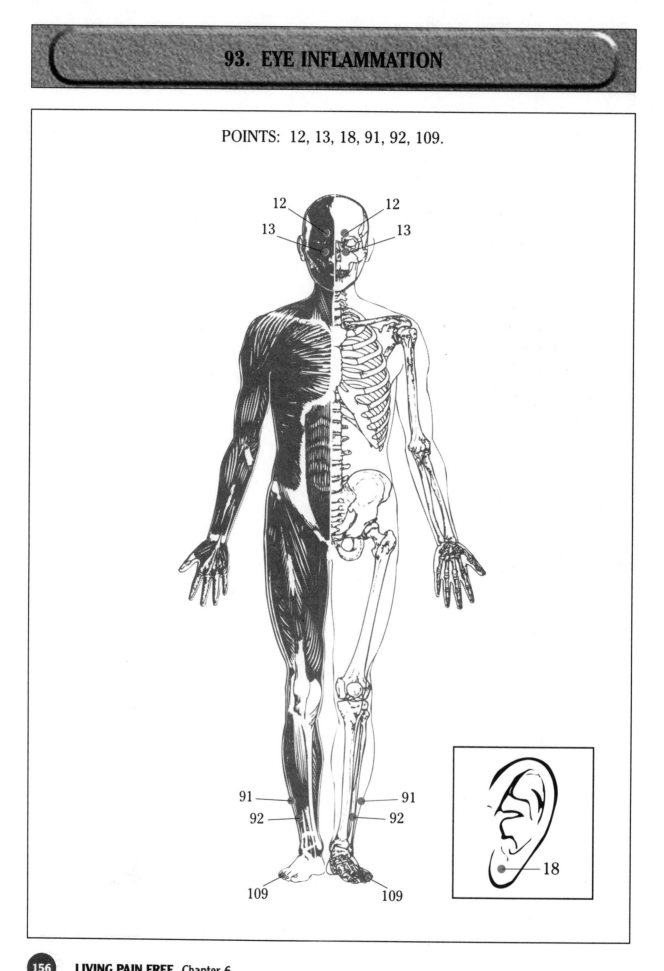

94. EYE INFECTIONS

POINTS: 7, 12, 13, 18, 44, 79, 91, 109, 110.

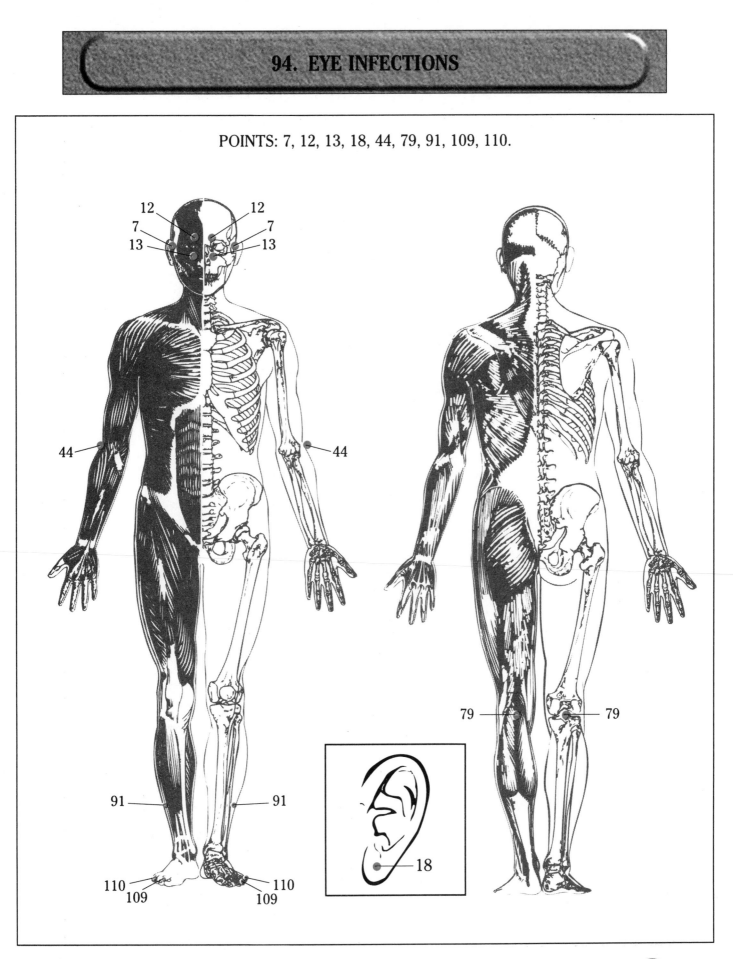

POINTS: 7, 9, 10, 12, 13, 18,

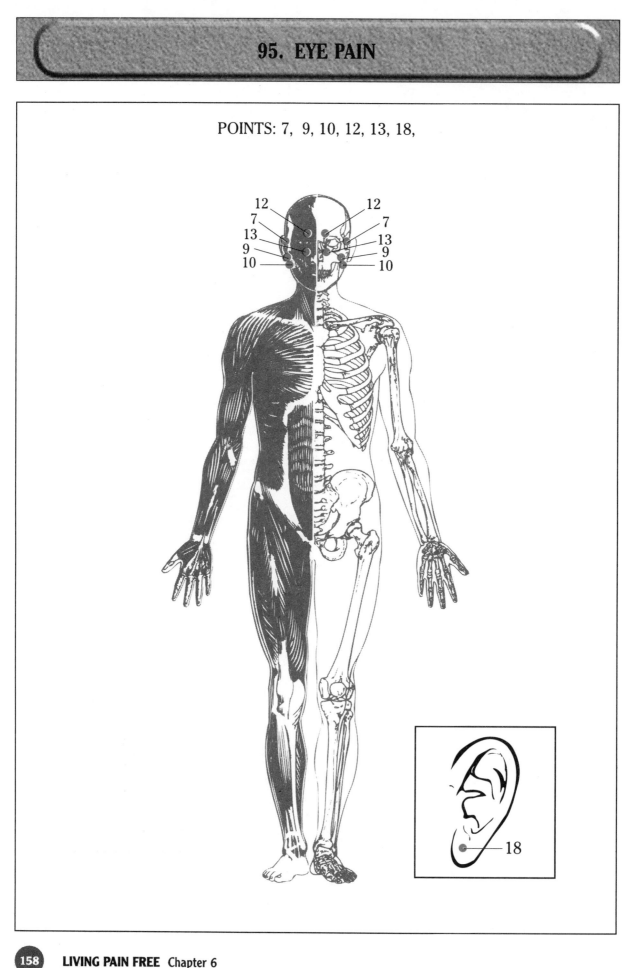

POINTS: 12, 13, 18, 91, 92, 109.

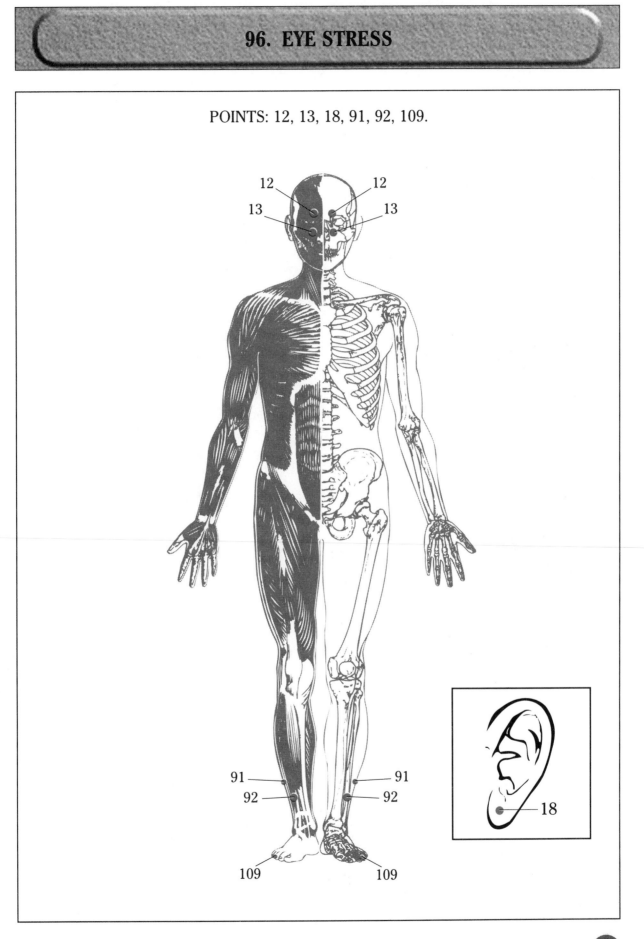

POINTS: 1, 15, 28, 34, 35, 52, 64, 70, 79, 99, 100, 101, 102, 107.

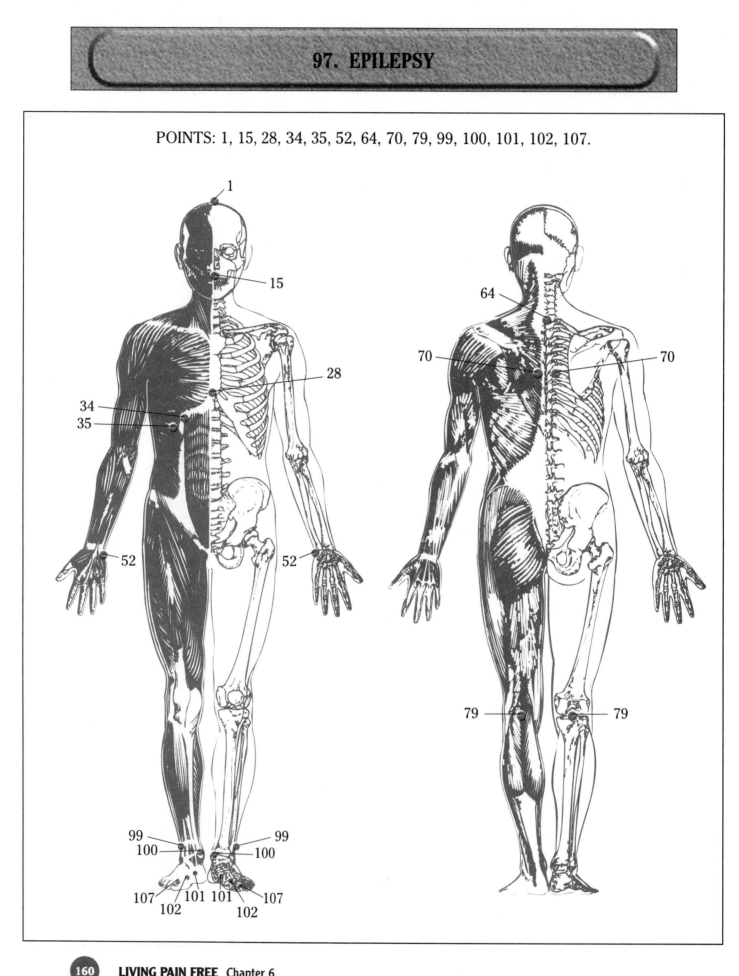

98. EPSTEIN-BARR VIRUS

POINTS: 24, 32, 44, 75, 79, 83, 95.

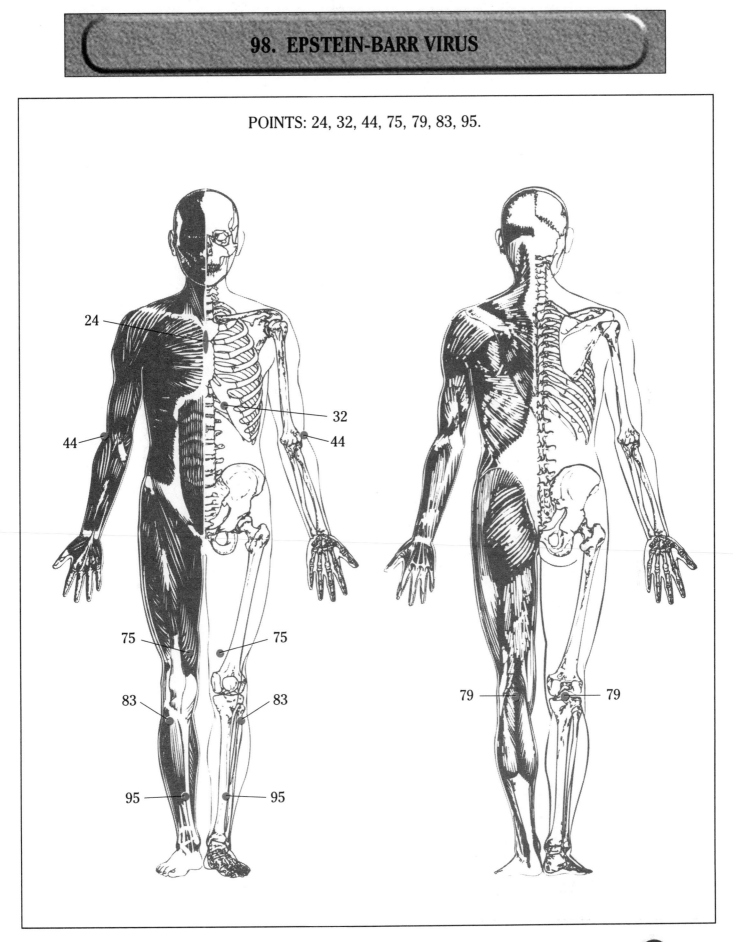

POINTS: 3, 21, 44, 64, 78, 94.

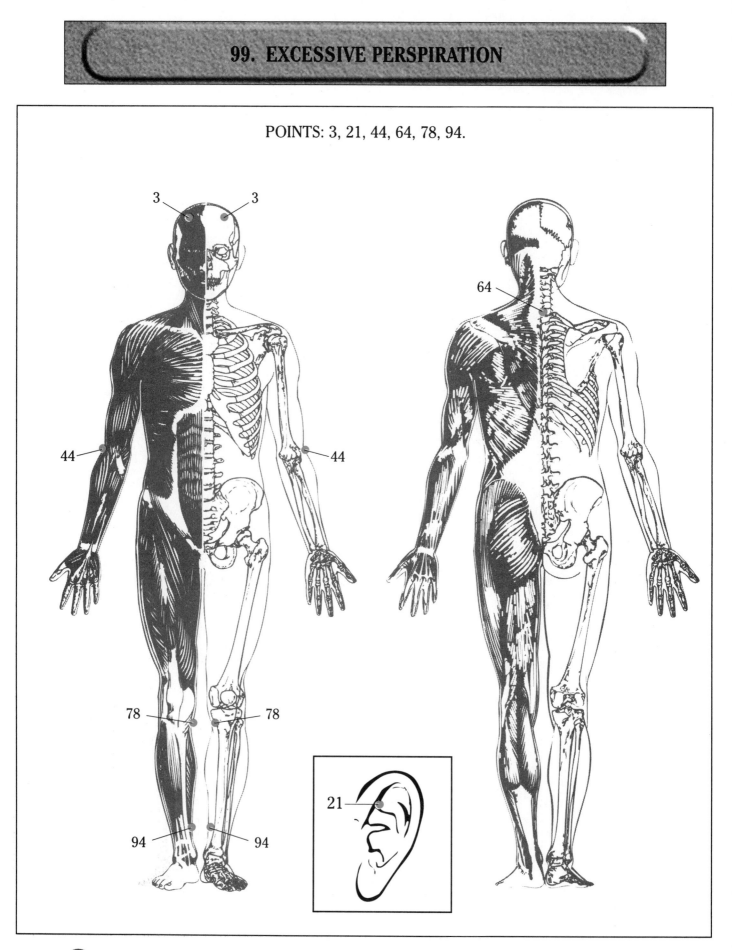

POINTS: 1, 15, 56, 58, 59, 61, 111.

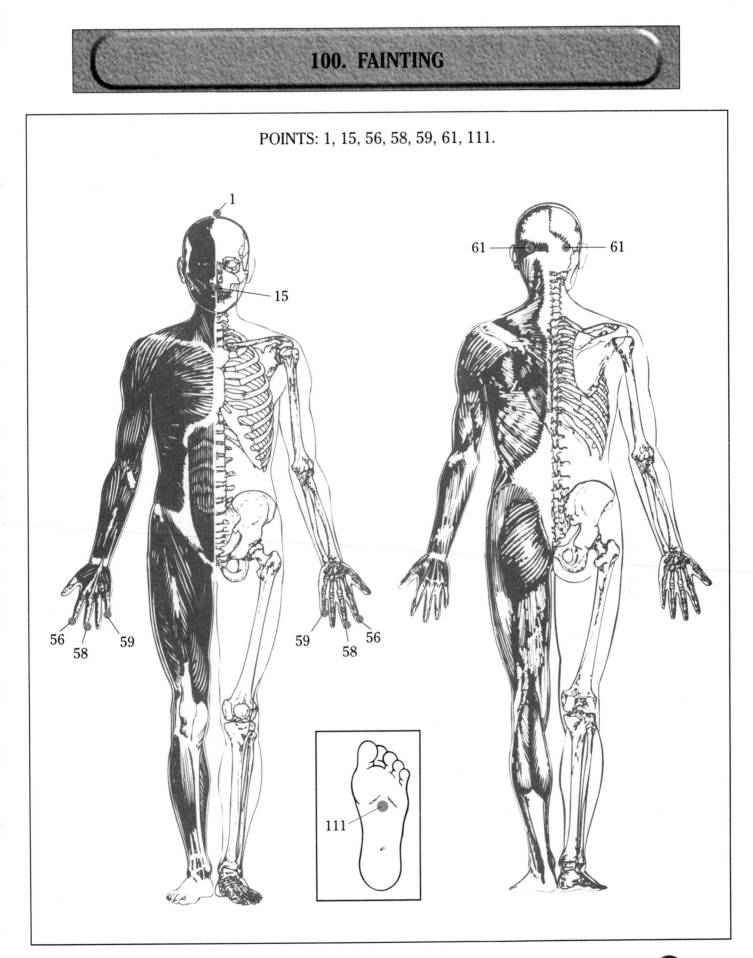

101. FEVER

POINTS: 44, 51, 53, 54, 58, 64, 71, 76, 104, 105, 108, 109, 111.

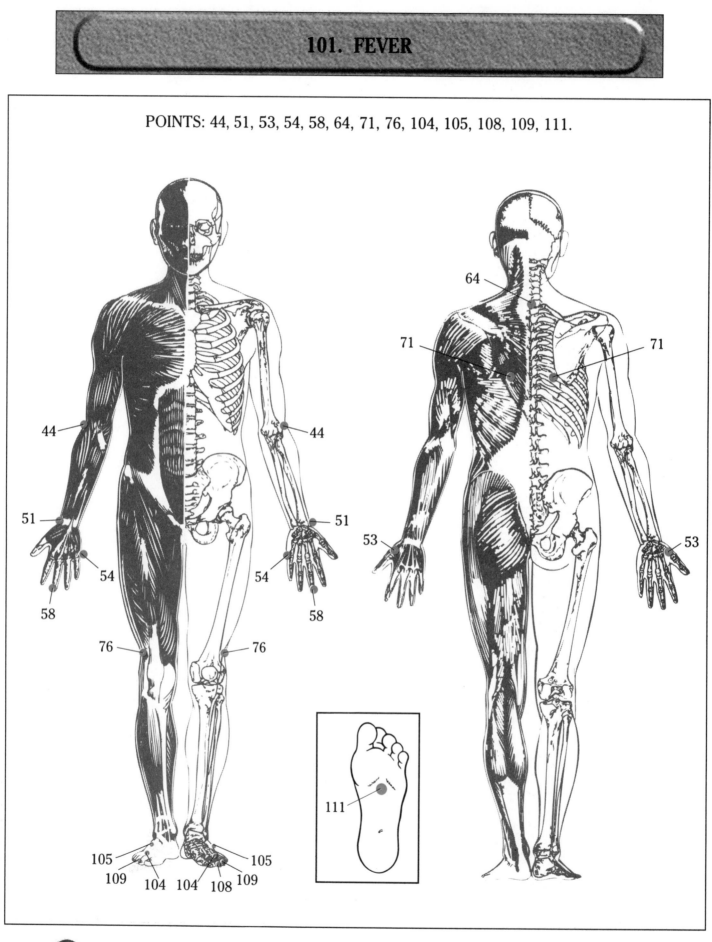

POINTS: 22, 27, 30, 39, 44, 46, 53, 75, 83, 96, 102.

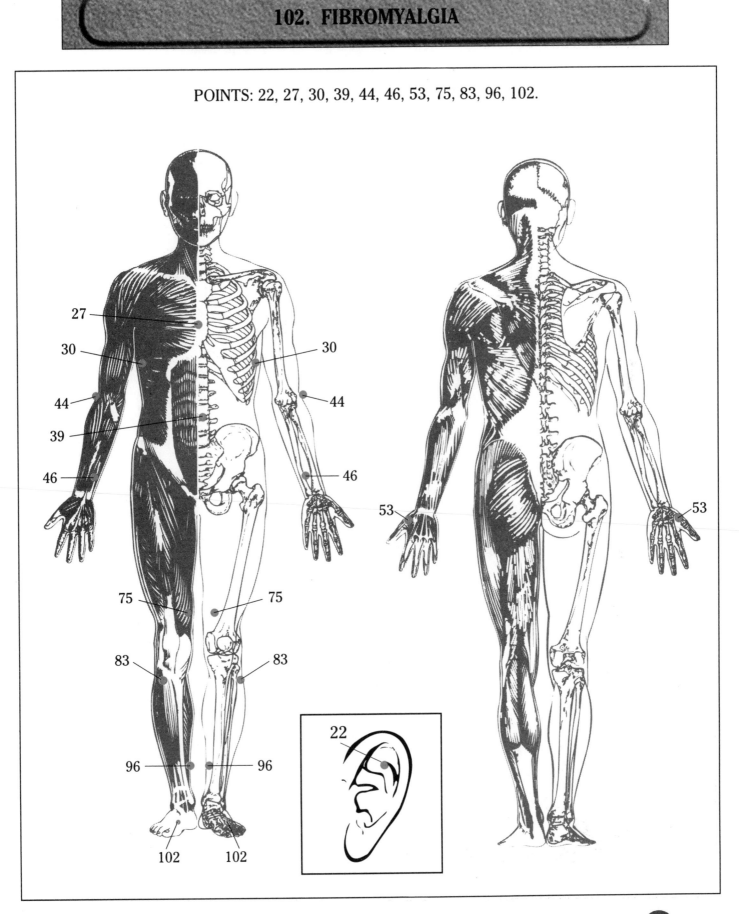

POINTS: 31, 36, 39, 46, 83, 101, 102.

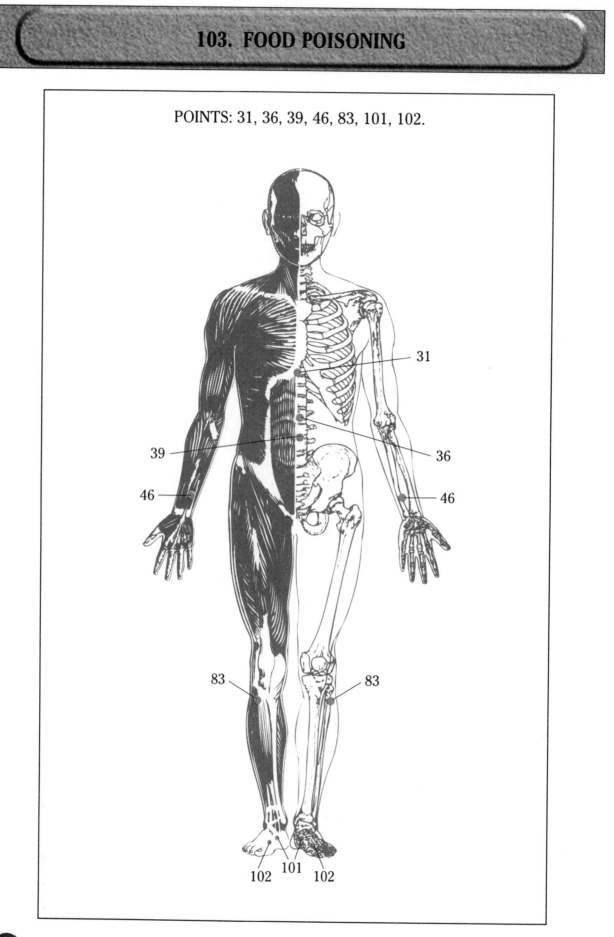

POINTS: 30, 44, 46, 83, 95, 96, 107.

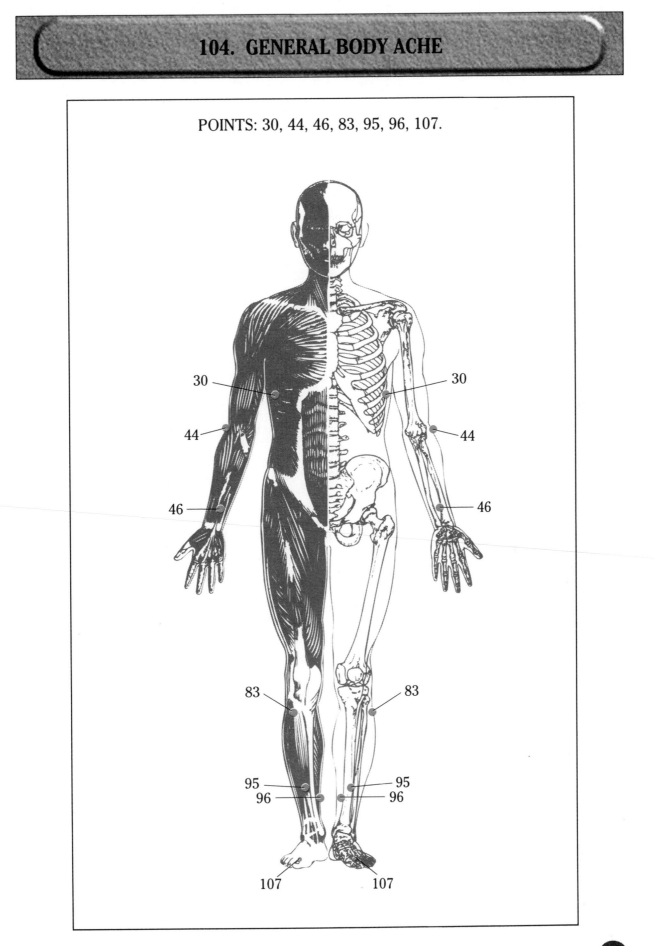

POINTS: 35, 38, 46, 49, 85, 86.

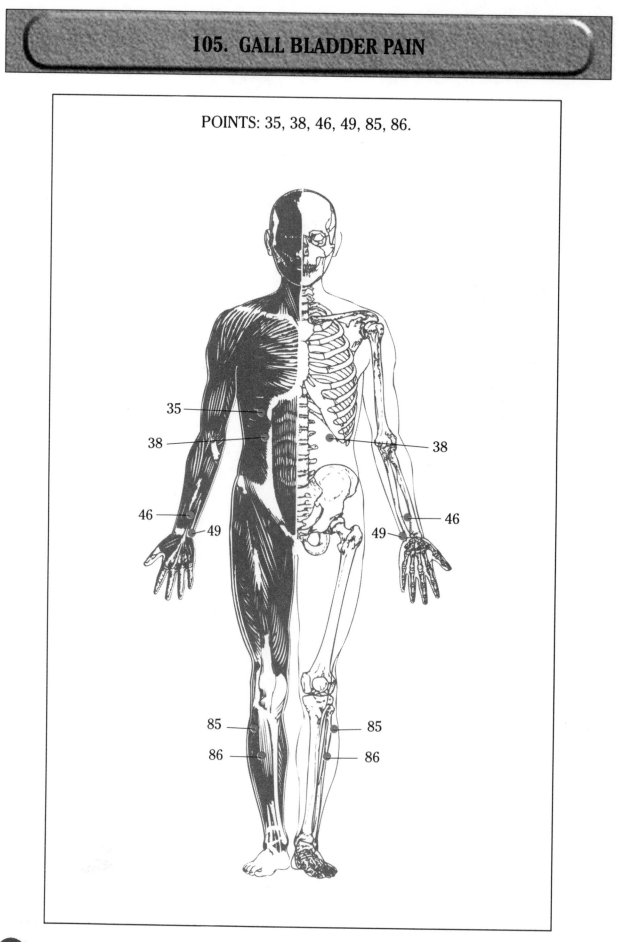

106. HEAT STROKE

POINTS: 1, 15, 44, 58, 65.

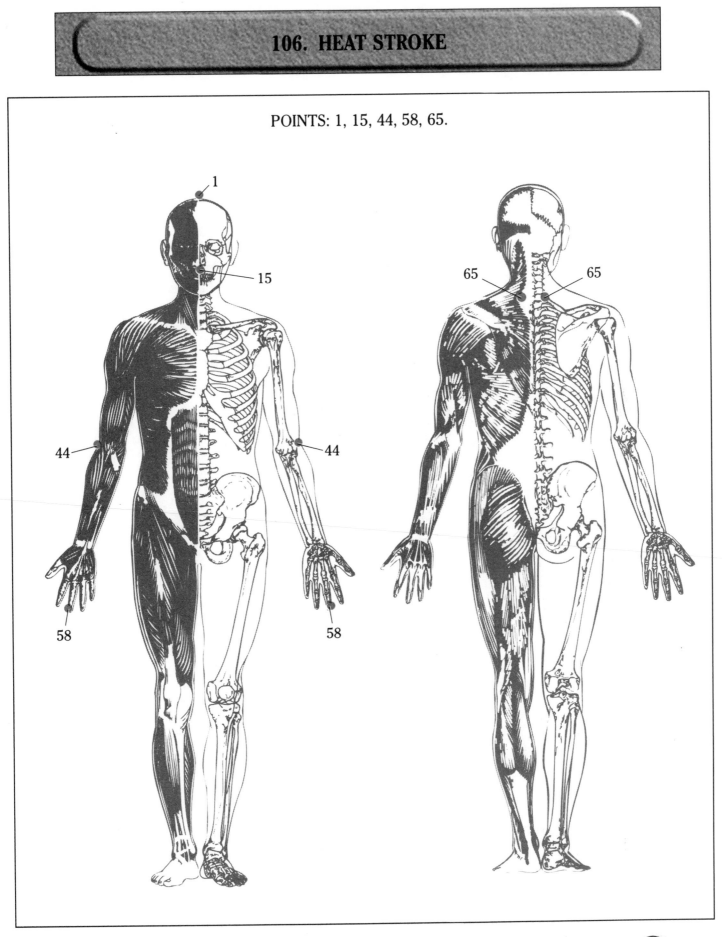

POINTS: 1, 47, 98, 99, 110, 111.

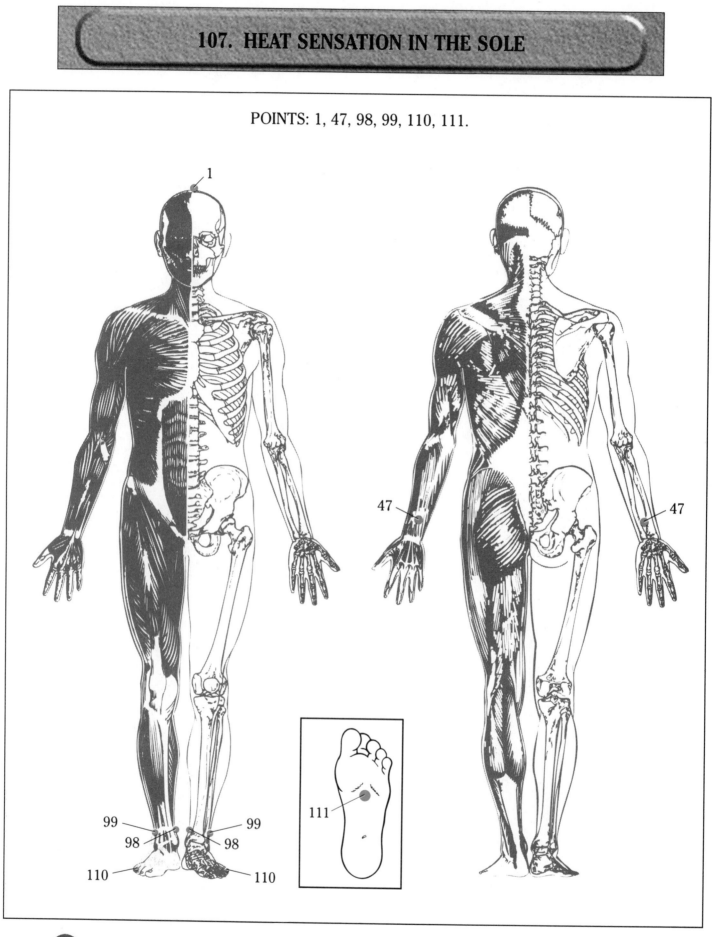

108. HEART IRREGULARITIES

POINTS: 1, 15, 46, 49, 58, 65.

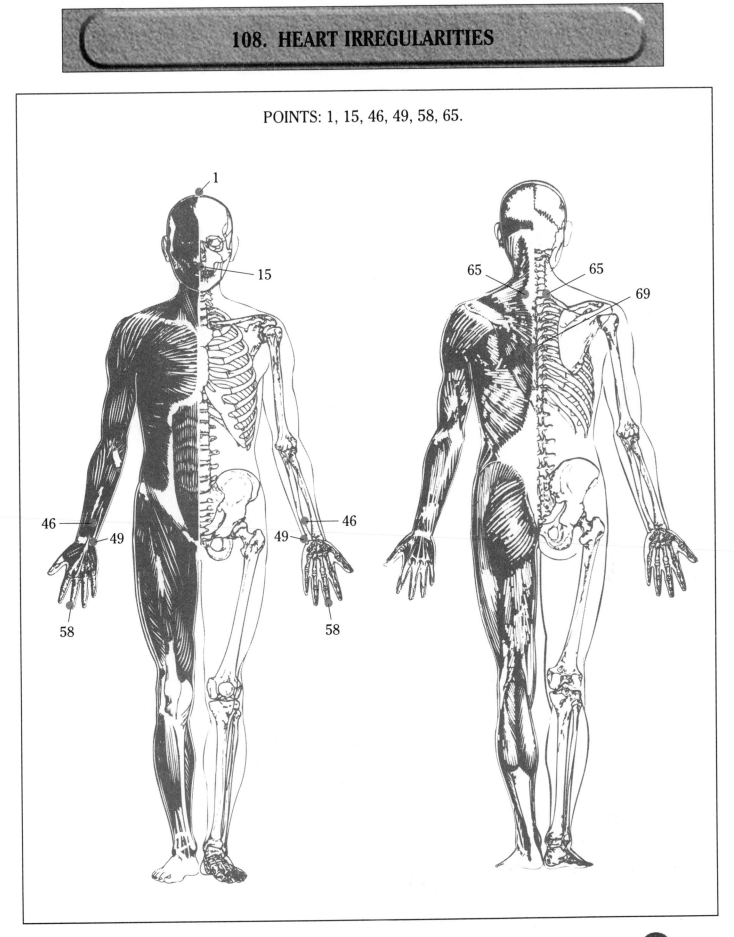

POINTS: 5, 31, 32, 33, 44, 46, 53, 76, 81, 83, 102, 106.

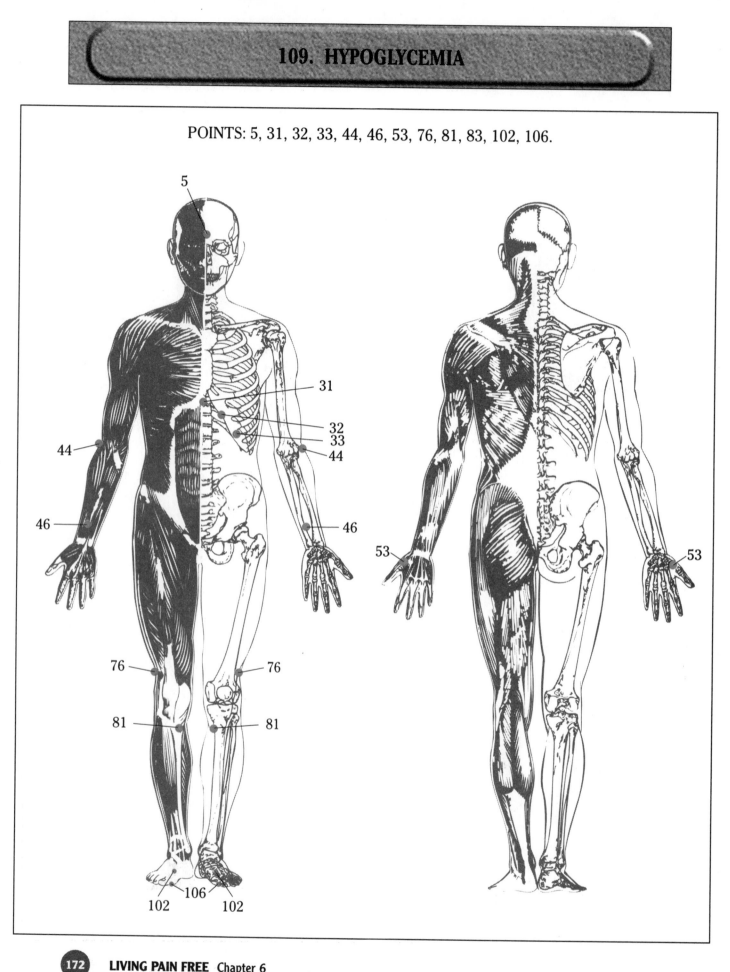

POINTS: 1, 2, 3, 5, 6, 10, 14, 15, 23, 63, 97.

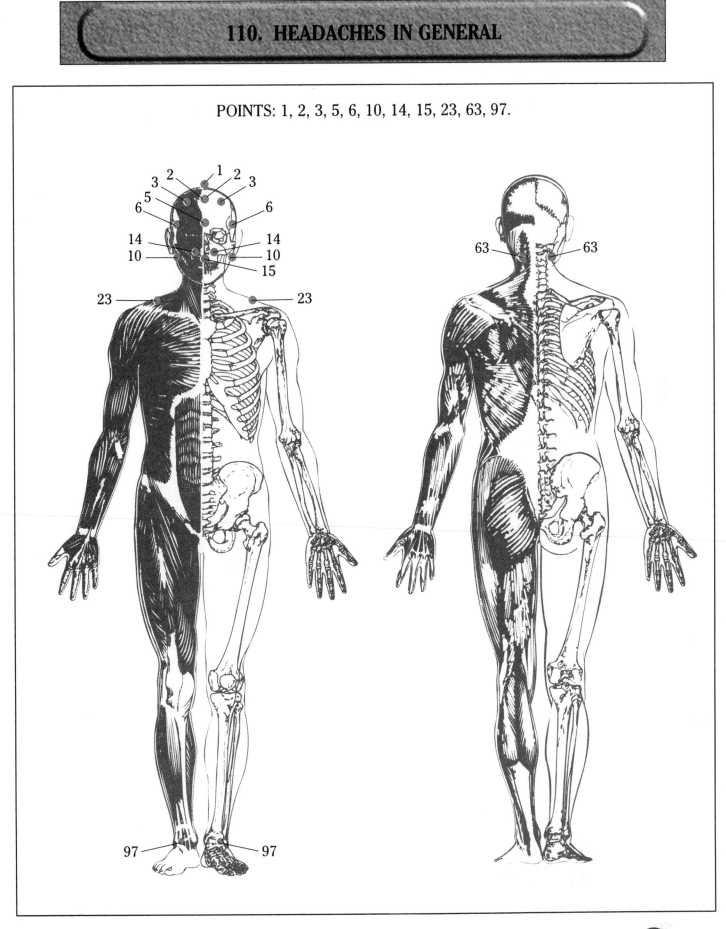

POINTS: 2, 3, 6, 12, 60, 63, 85, 103.

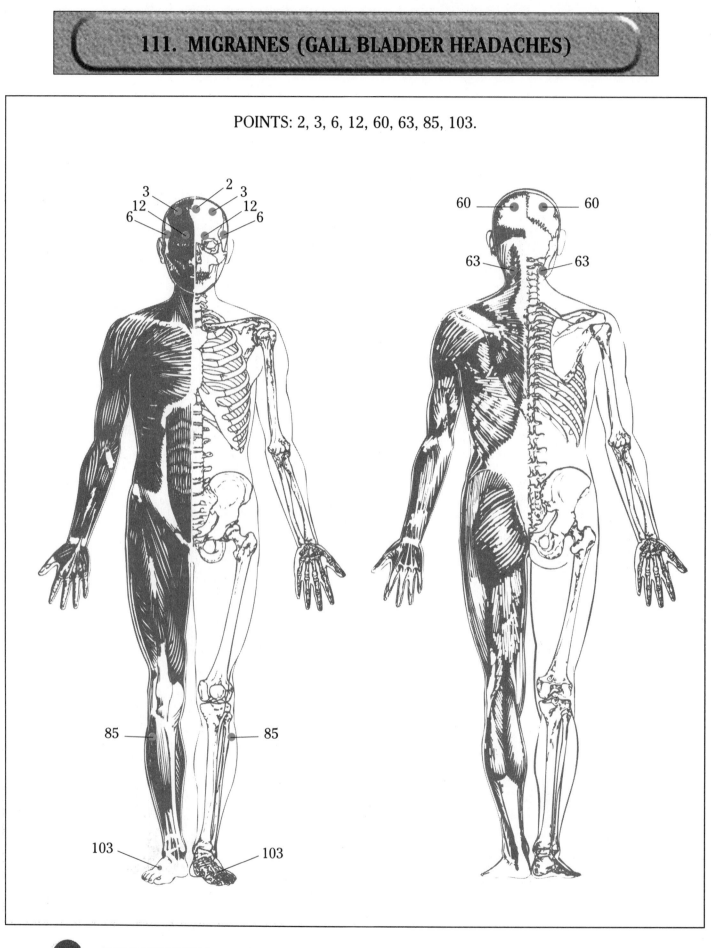

112. MIGRAINES (LIVER HEADACHES)

POINTS: 1, 2, 3, 7, 60, 63, 85, 95, 103.

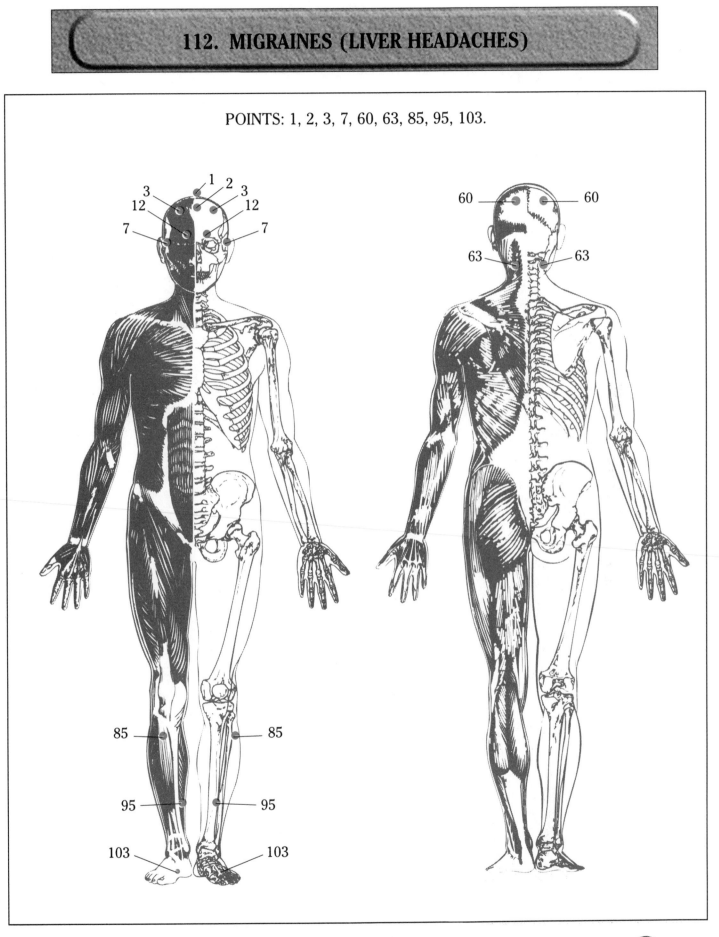

POINTS: 2, 3, 4, 5, 12, 31, 44, 53, 83, 87, 97.

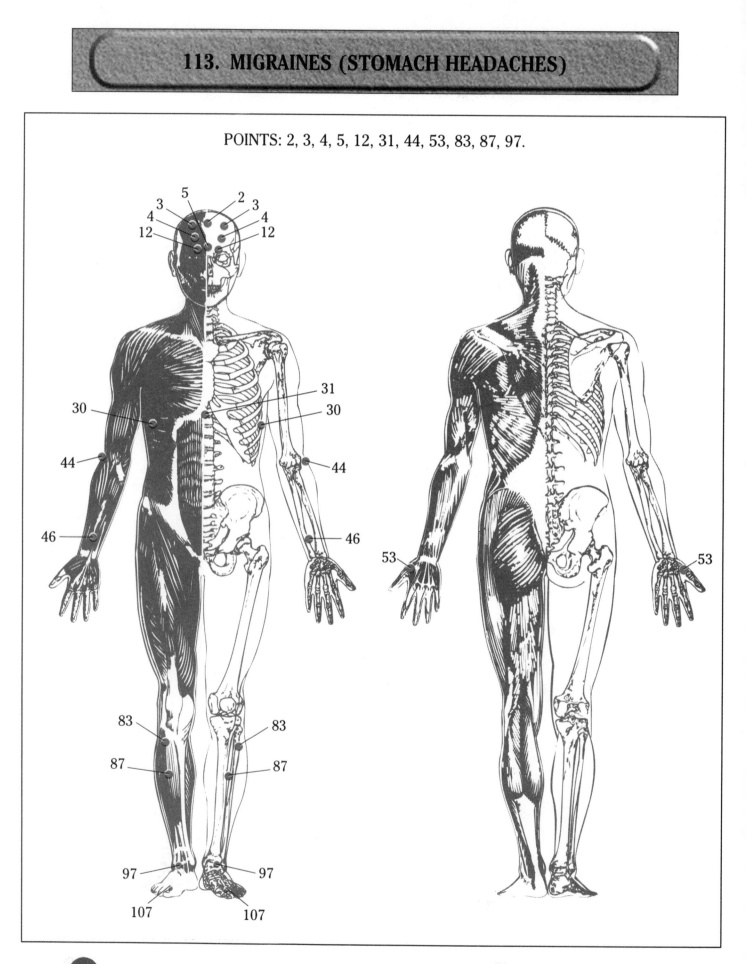

114. MIGRAINES (BLADDER HEADACHES)

POINTS: 1, 12, 14, 44, 53, 64, 63, 60, 79, 94, 98, 99.

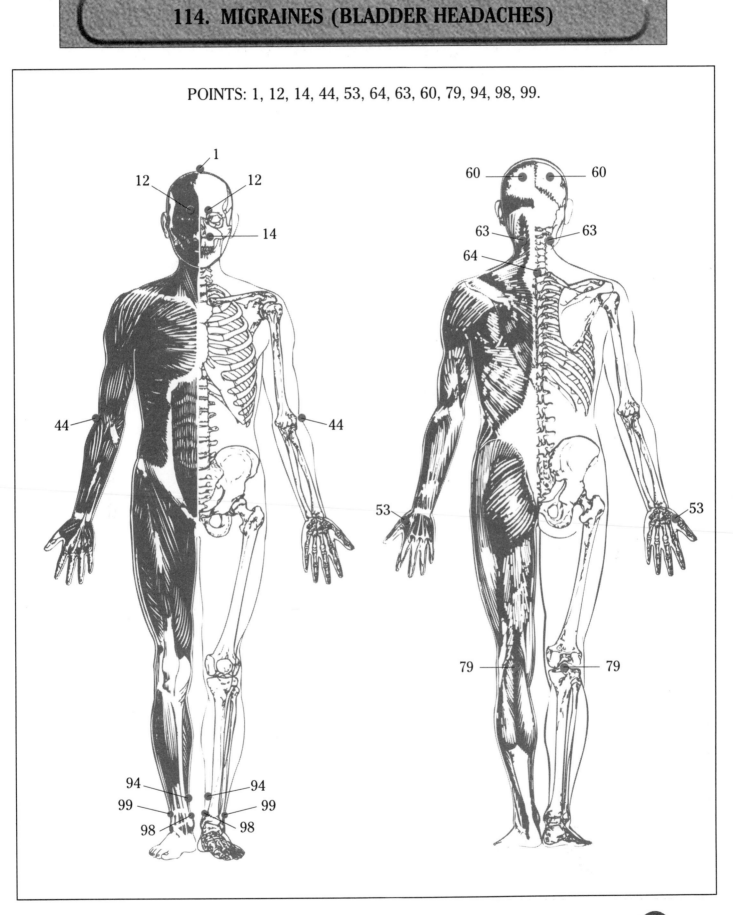

POINTS: 28, 31, 32, 33, 46, 83.

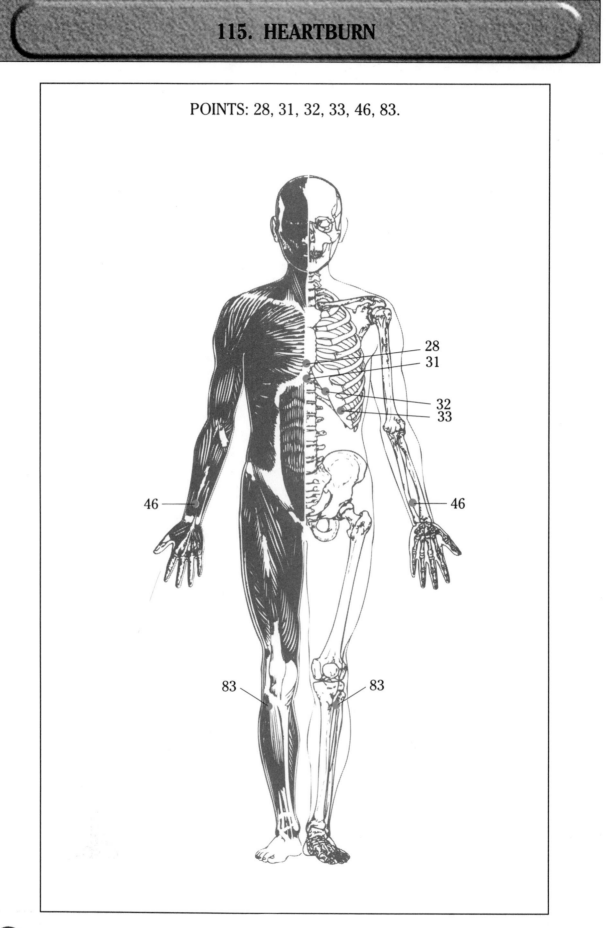

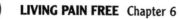

116. HIGH BLOOD PRESSURE

POINTS: 1, 44, 53, 62, 63, 64, 83, 93, 95, 102.

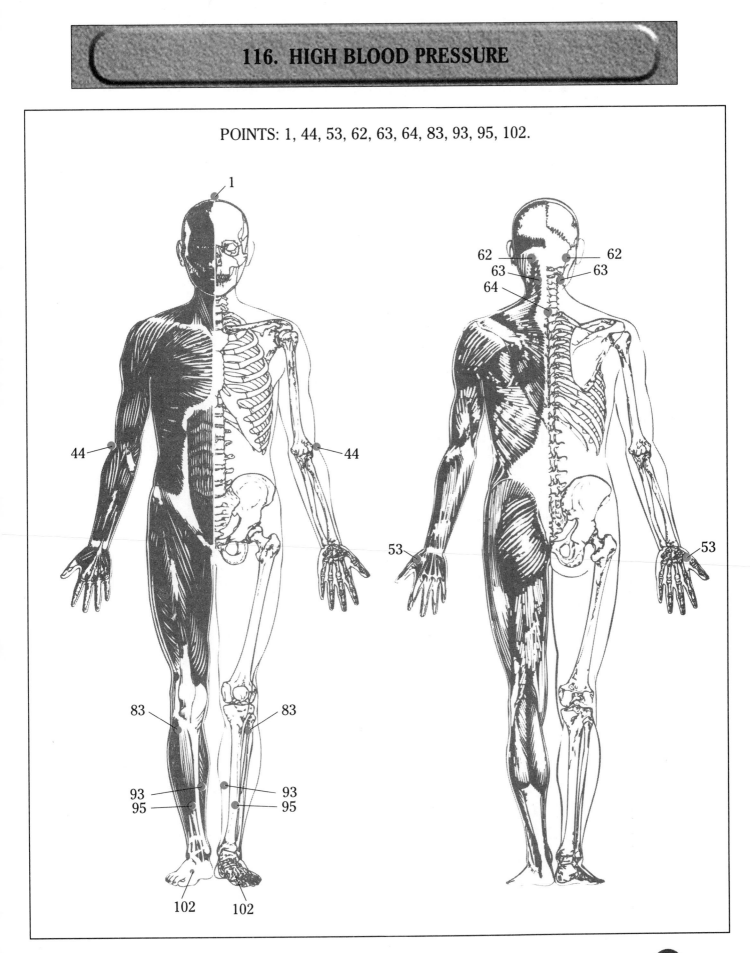

117. HIVES

POINTS: 22, 38, 44, 46, 53, 75, 79.

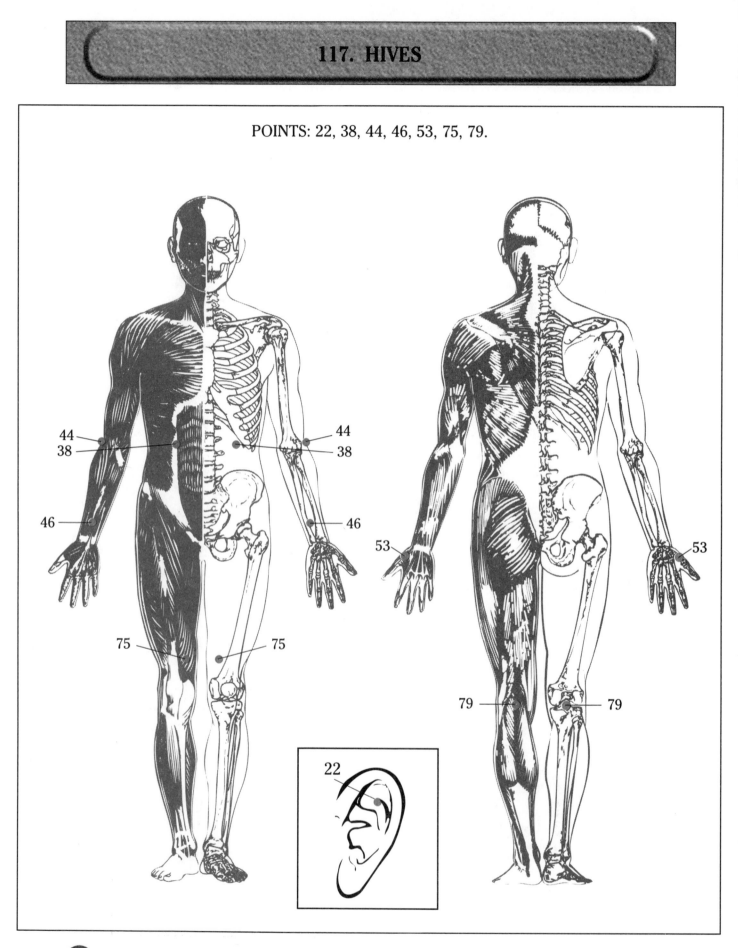

118. INDIGESTION

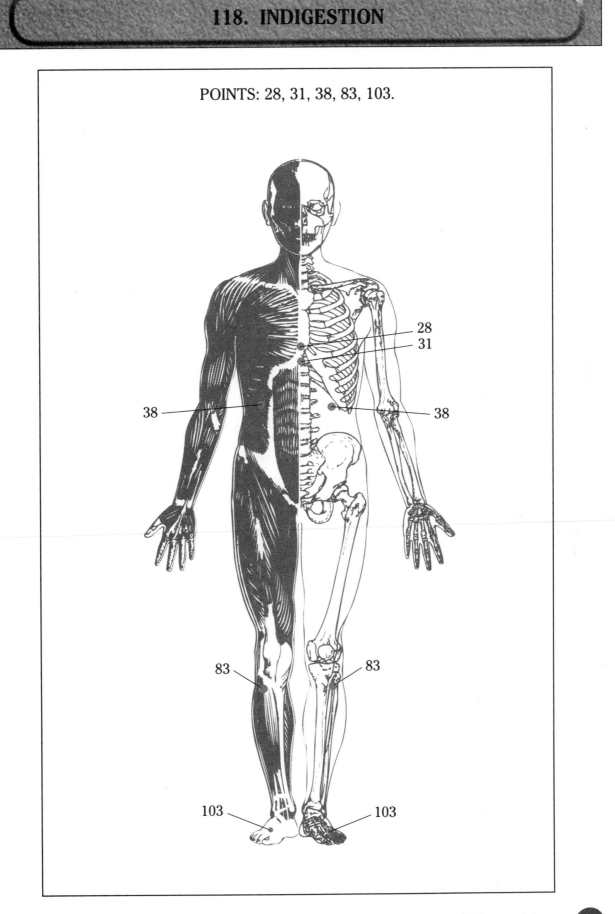

POINTS: 28, 31, 38, 83, 103.

28
31
38
38
83
83
103
103

POINTS: 1, 48, 49, 62, 78, 81, 94, 98, 100.

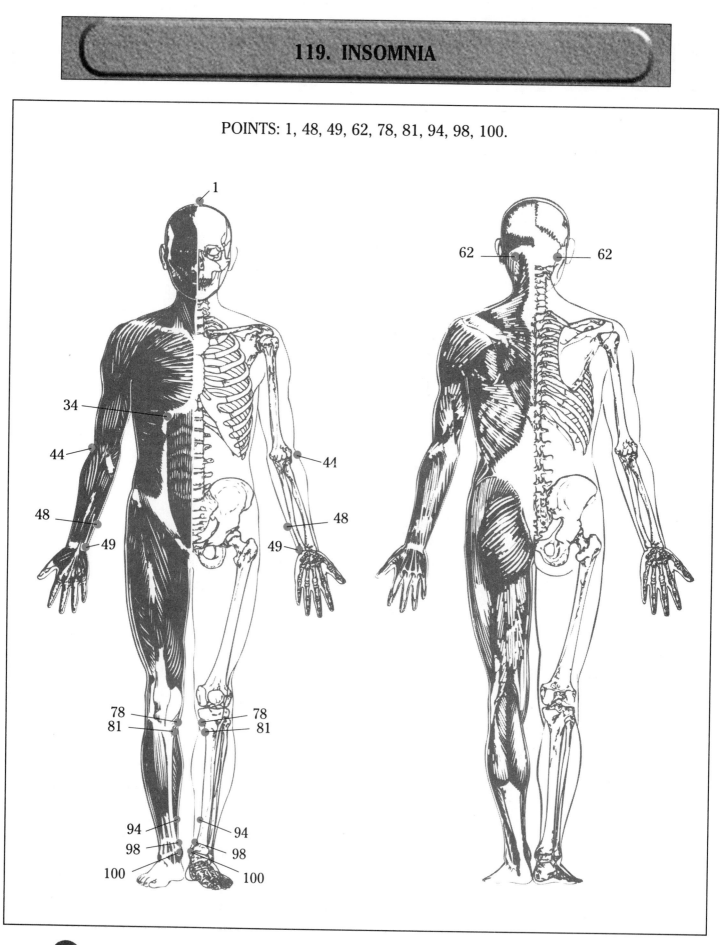

120. LARYNGITIS

POINTS: 24, 27, 55, 111.

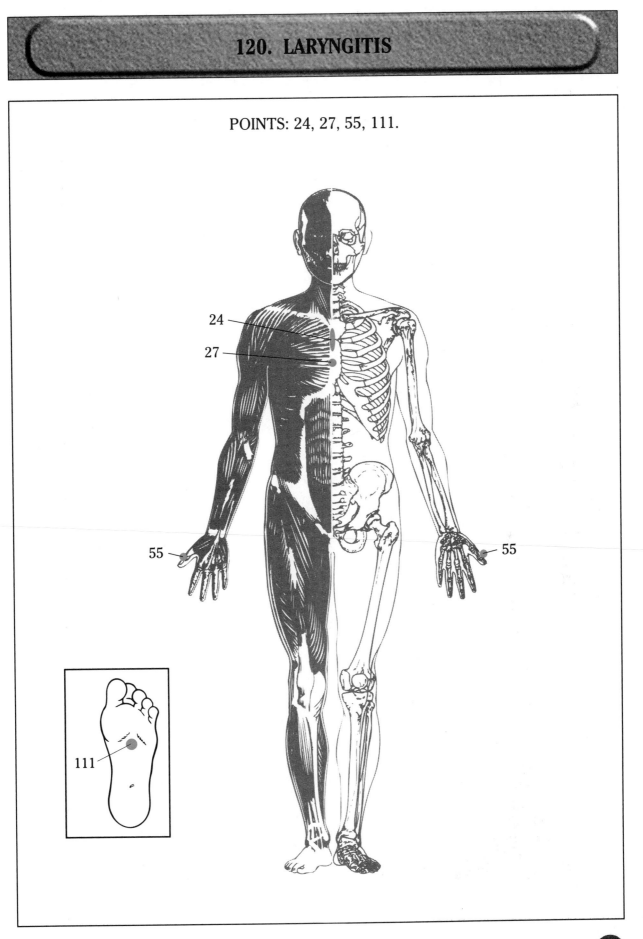

POINTS: 31, 36, 40, 87, 88, 96, 101.

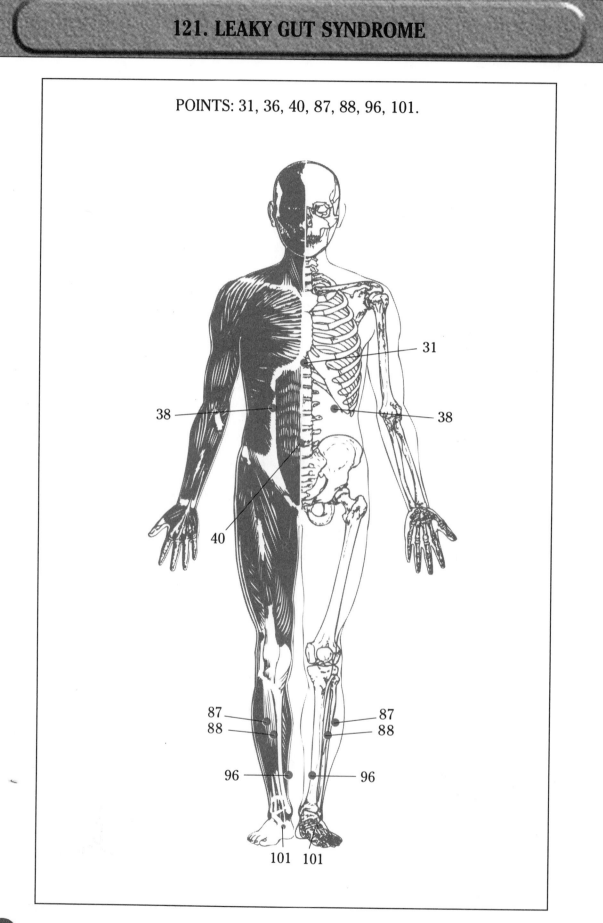

POINTS: 1, 15, 27, 39, 66, 71, 83, 94, 95, 102.

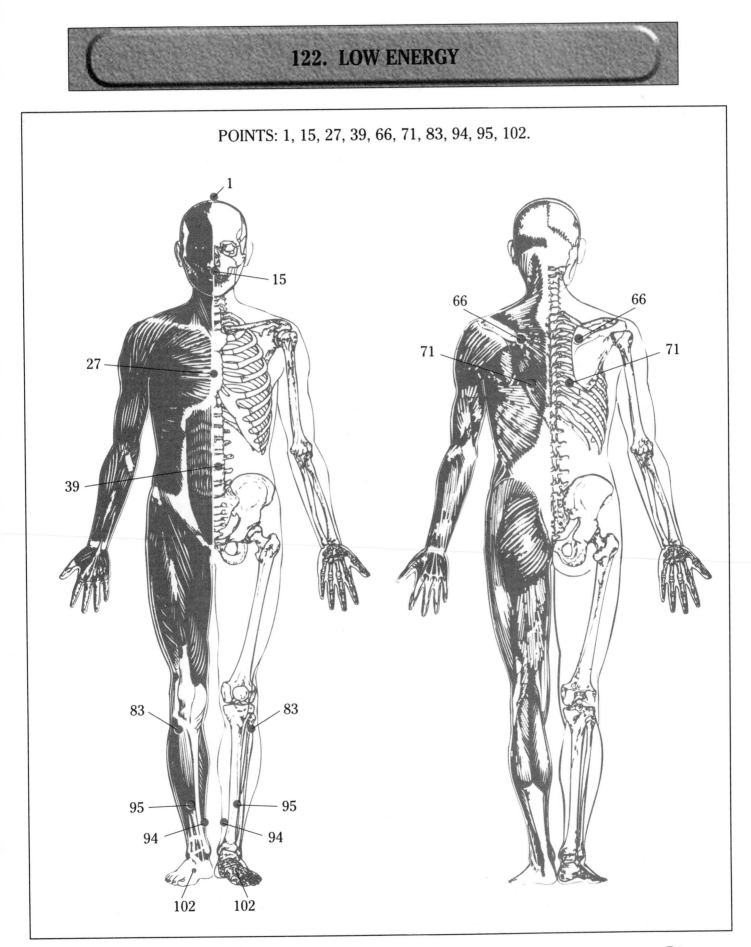

123. MENSTRUATION TROUBLE (P.M.S.)

POINTS: 15, 40, 46, 53, 75, 82, 96, 102.

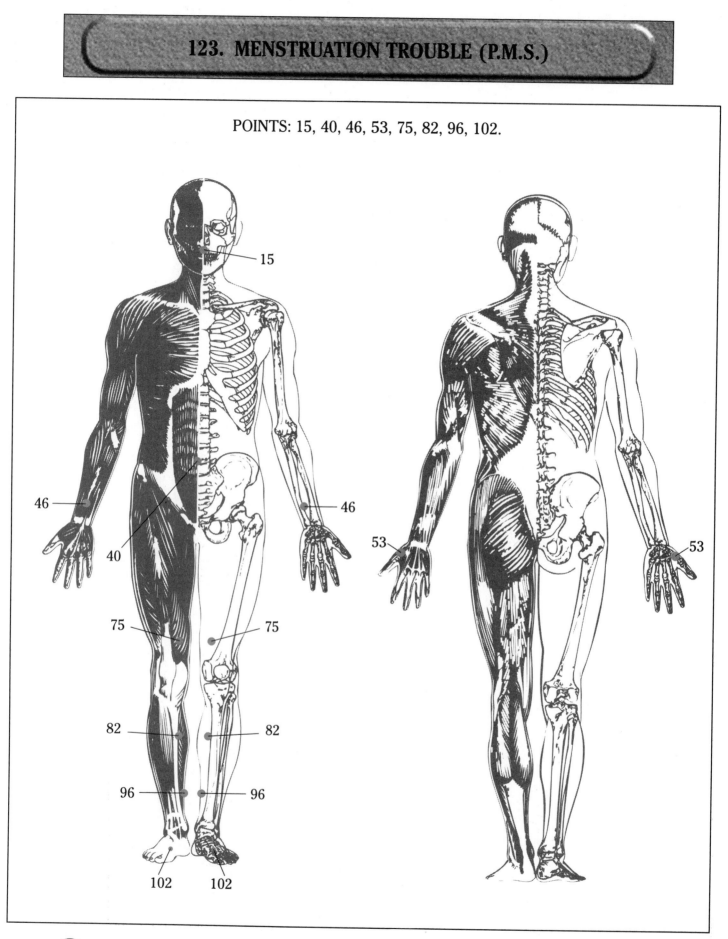

POINTS: 15, 31, 46.

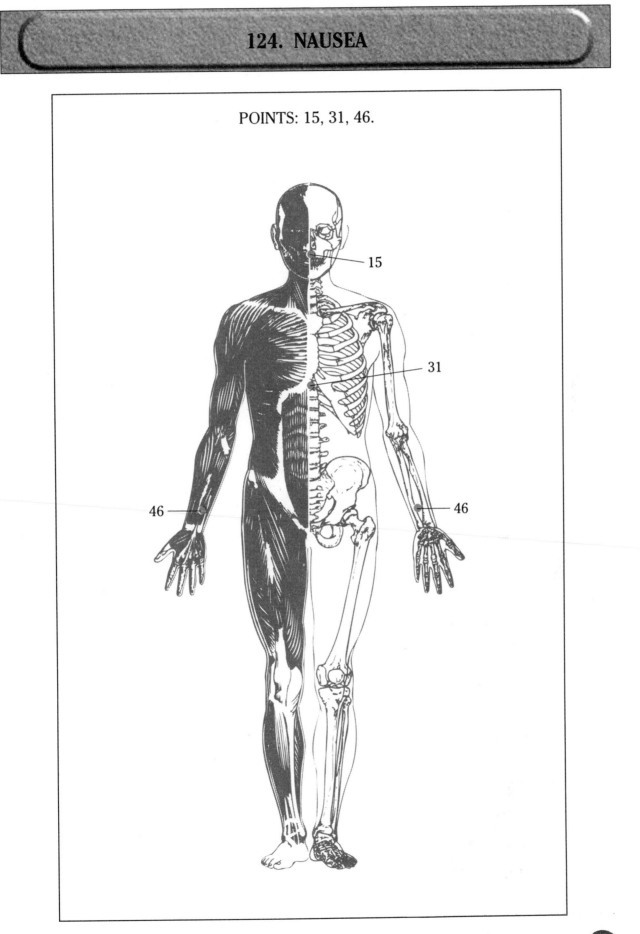

POINTS: 1, 5, 46, 49, 48.

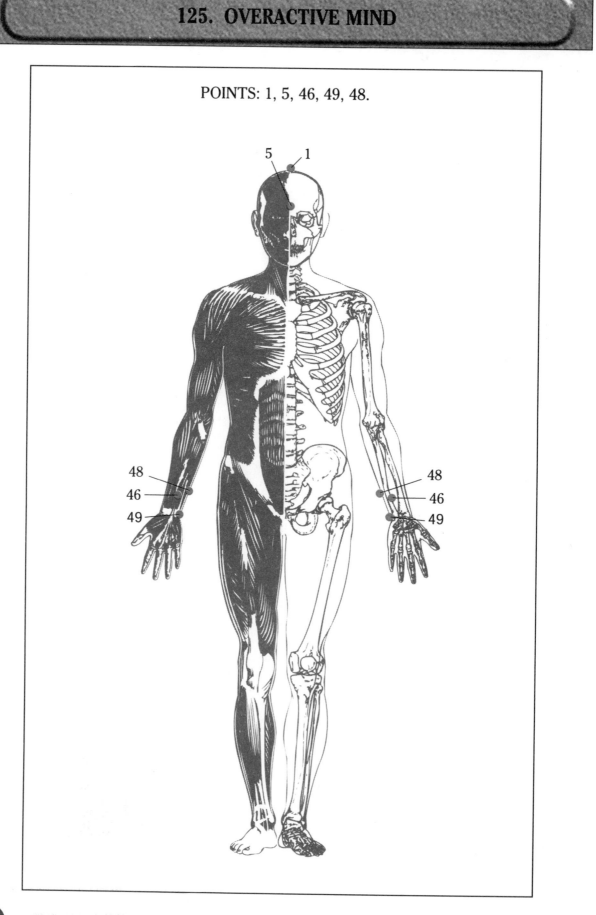

POINTS: 1, 15, 27, 39, 71, 83, 88, 95, 102.

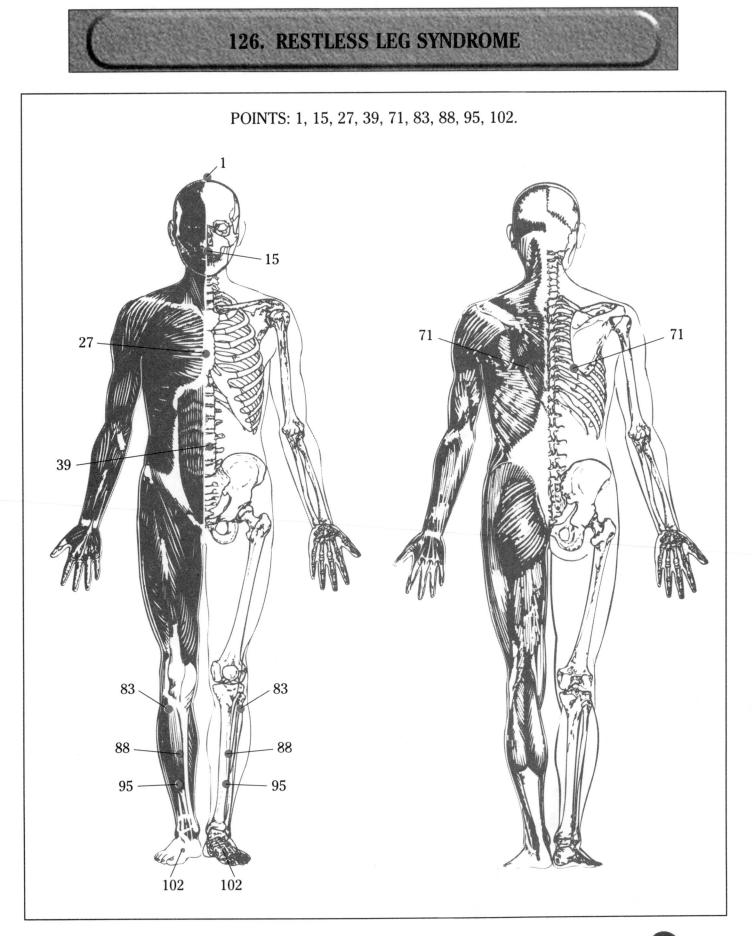

127. SCIATIC NEURALGIA

POINTS: 14, 15, 42, 46, 57, 72, 76, 79.

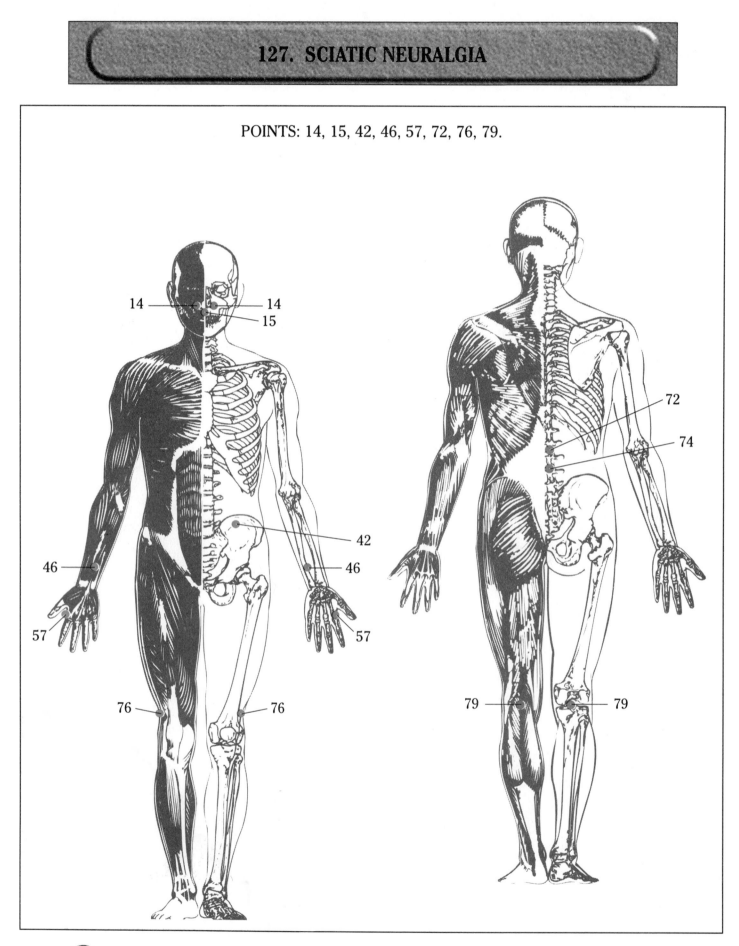

128. SHORTNESS OF BREATH

POINTS: 15, 20, 24, 25, 26, 27, 28, 31, 38, 39, 45, 50, 53, 102,

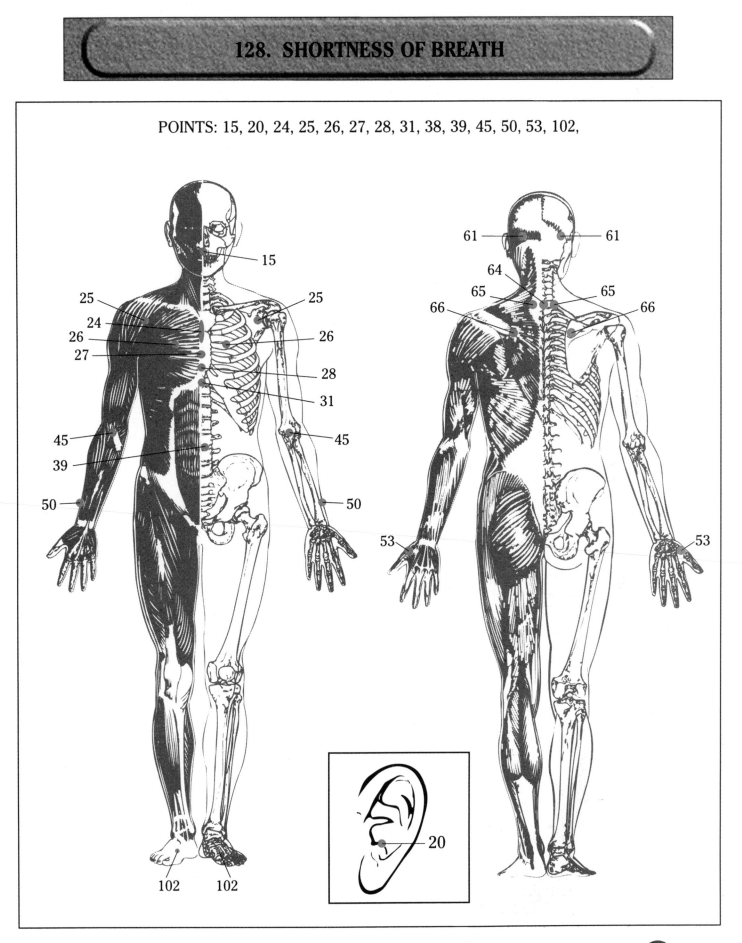

POINTS: 14, 44, 53, 55, 102.

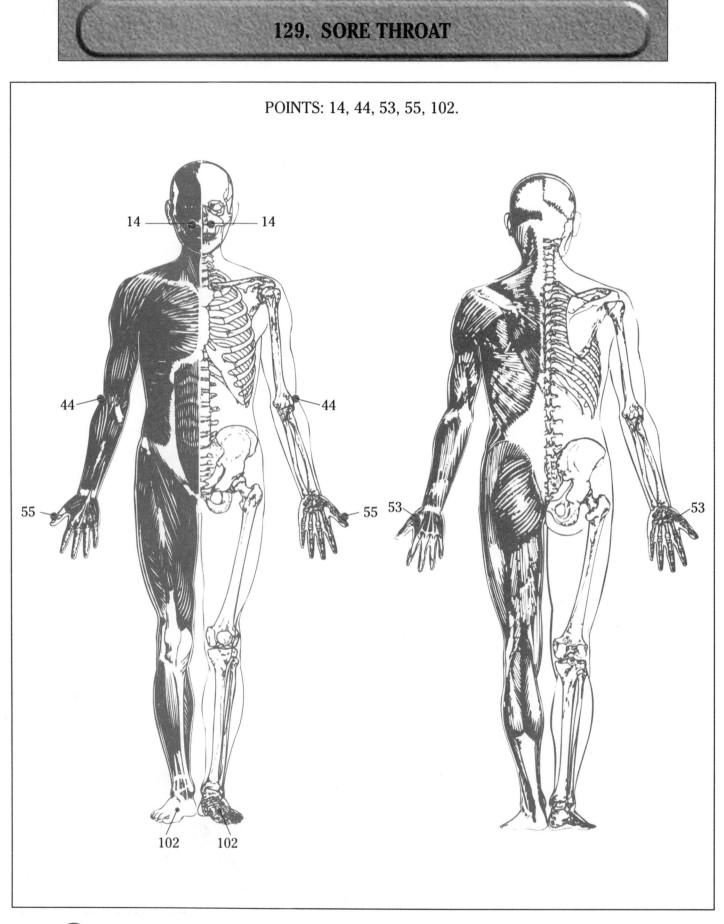

POINTS: 9, 47, 53, 98, 99, 103.

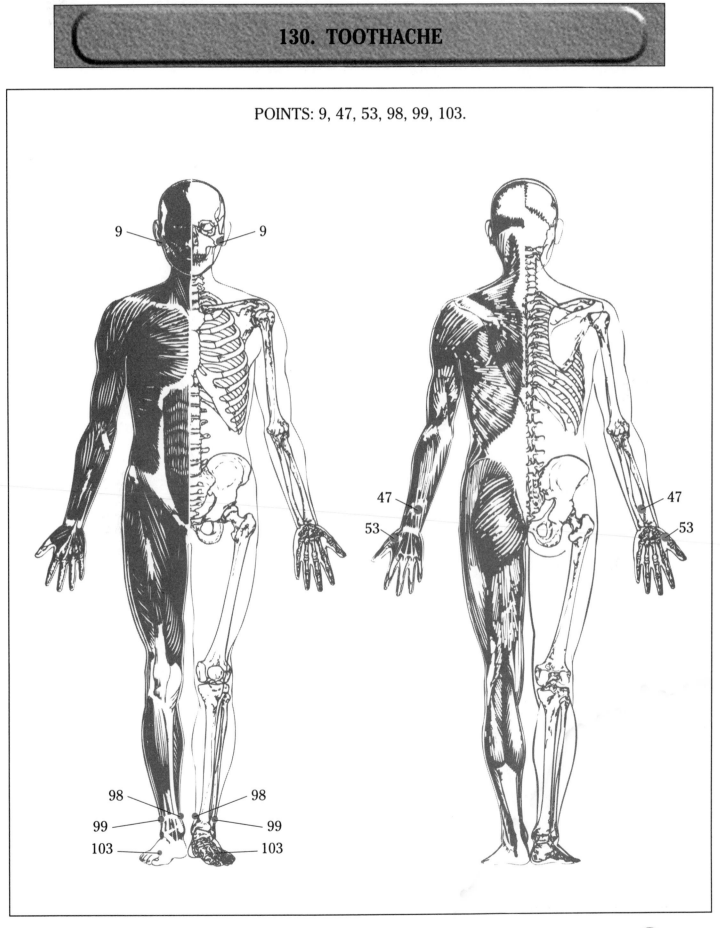

POINTS: 26, 27, 34, 35, 46, 49, 52.

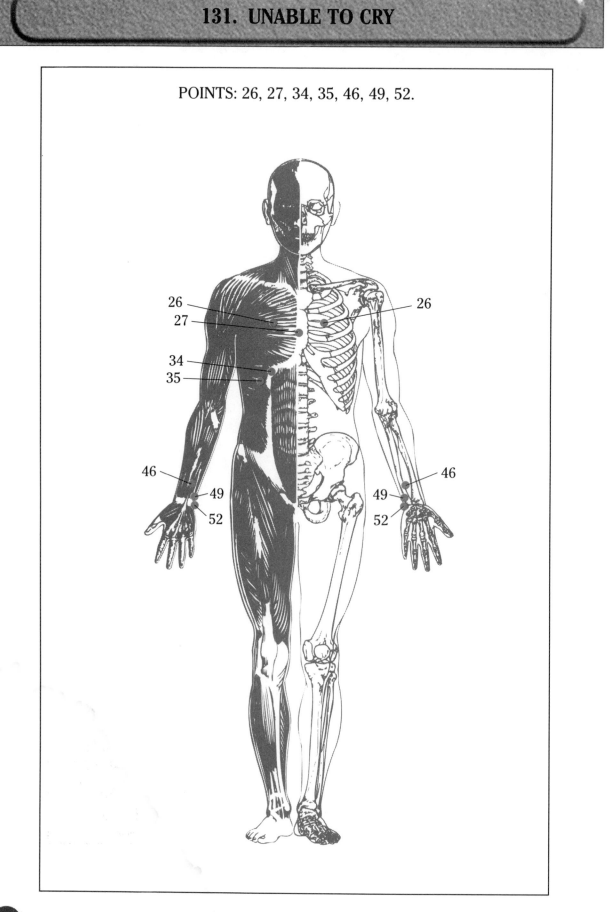

132. NERVOUSNESS OF ALL KINDS

POINTS: 21, 22, 27, 31, 46, 49, 52.

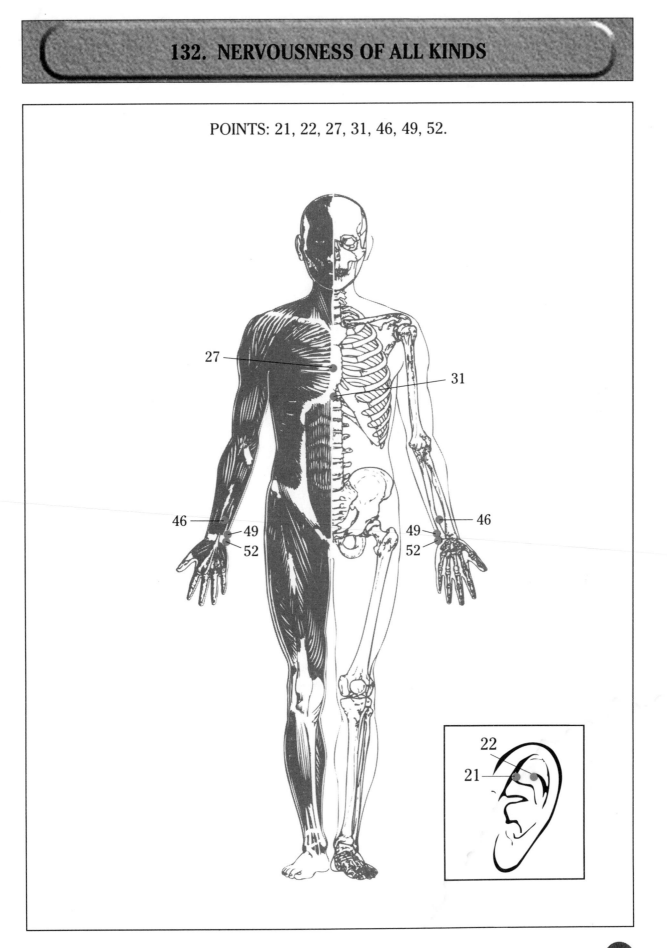

Bibliography

1. Say Good Bye To Illness
by Devi S. Nambudripad, Delta Publishing, Buena Park, CA
1990, 1993

2. NAET Guide Book
by Devi S. Nambudripad, Delta Publishing, Buena Park, CA
1994, 1996

3. Essentials of Chinese Acupuncture - compiled
by Beijing College of Traditional Chinese Medicine, Shanghai College of Traditional Chinese Medicine, Nanjing College of Traditional Chinese Medicine, The Acupuncture Institute of the Academy of Traditional Chinese Medicine, Beijing, China: Foreign Language Press,
1981 (1st Edition)

4. Introduction to Chinese Acupuncture
by Kwong-Ming, Ma-Hong Kong, China: The Standard Chinese Medicine, Acupuncture Healing Center,
1976

5. Acupuncture: A Comprehensive Text
Shanghai College of Traditional Medicine. translated and edited by John O'Connor and Dan Bensky, Chicago, Illinois, Eastland Press
1981

6. Food, Nutrition and Diet Therapy
M.V. Krause and L.K. Mahan, W.V. Saunders Company, Philadelphia, PA
1979

7. Function A Human Anatomy
James E. Crouch, 2nd Edition, Lea & Febiger, Philadelphia, PA
1972

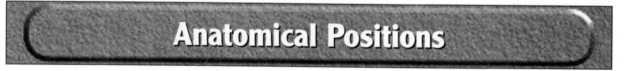

Anatomical Positions

Posterior ....Refers to back
Dorsal ....Refers to back
Anterior ....Refers to front of the body
Ventral ....Refers to front of the body.
Superior........................Refers to upper or higher part of body.
Inferior.........................Means the lower part of the body.
Medial ....Area near the midline of the body.
Lateral ....Area away from the midline of the body.
Distal ....Area away from the heart
Proximal ....Area closer to the heart.

If anyone would like to get more information about the human anatomy, please read Gray's Anatomy or Functional Human anatomy in any Library or book store.

Index

	Page	Diagram Page
ABDOMINAL BLOATING	33	64
ABDOMINAL PAIN	33	65
ABDOMINAL PAINS DUE TO OVEREATING	33	66
ABDOMINAL SPASMS	33	67
ACNE	34	72
ACUPRESSURE	10	
ACUPUNCTURE	10	
ACUTE APPENDICITIS	34	70
ACUTE VIRAL INFECTION	34	69
ADDICTION TO DRUGS	34	73
ADDICTION TO FOOD	34	73
ADHD	34	71
ANGER	35	4
ANGIONEUROTIC EDEMA	35	75
ANOREXIA NERVOSA	35	76
ANXIETY ATTACKS	35	77
ARTHRITIS OF THE ANKLES AND TOES	37	85
ARTHRITIS OF THE ELBOW	36	80
ARTHRITIS OF THE FINGERS	35	78
ARTHRITIS OF THE HAND	35	79
ARTHRITIS OF THE HIP JOINT	36	83
ARTHRITIS OF THE KNEE	36	84
ARTHRITIS OF THE SHOULDER	36	81
ARTHRITIS OF THE WRIST	36	82
ASCITES	38	89
ASTHMA	38	90
BACTERIAL INFECTION	38	94
BLEEDING FROM THE EYES	39	97
BLEEDING FROM THE GUMS	39	95
BLEEDING FROM THE MOUTH	39	98
BLEEDING FROM THE MUCOUS MEMBRANES	39	99
BLEEDING FROM THE NOSE	39	96
BLEEDING FROM THE RECTUM	40	105
BLEEDING FROM THE STOMACH	40	100
BLOCKAGE OF THE SINUSES	41	108
BLOOD DISORDERS	40	101
BLOOD IN THE STOOL	40	102
BLOOD IN THE URINE	40	103
BLURRED VISION	41	109
BRAIN FOG	41	110
BRONCHITIS	42	112
BULIMIA	42	113
BURNING FEET	41	107
BUTTERFLY SENSATION OR NERVOUS STOMACH	42	106
CARDIAC ARREST AND RESPIRATORY ARREST	42	115
CELIAC SPRUE	43	117
CHEMICAL SENSITIVITY	43	118
CHEST PAINS OR CARDIAC PAINS	43	116
CHI	11	
CHOKING WHILE YOU TALK TO STRANGERS (SHYNESS)	44	123
CHRONIC FATIGUE SYNDROME	44	124
COLD LIMBS	44	122
COLD SORES	45	127
COLIC	33	
COLITIS	44	126
COMA OR SEMICONSCIOUSNESS	44	125
COMMON COLD	45	128

	Page	Diagram Page
CONNECTIVE TISSUE DISORDERS	59	
CONSTANT ALLERGIC REACTIONS	59	24
CONSTIPATION	44	121
CONVULSIONS	45	129
COUGH	45	130
CRAMPS IN THE LEGS	45	131
CRAMPS IN THE LOWER ABDOMEN	45	132
CROHN'S DISEASE/IRRITABLE BOWELS	46	133
CRYING SPELLS	46	134
DEAFNESS AND RINGING IN THE EAR	46	135
DECREASED WHITE BLOOD CELL COUNT	59	
DELAYED MENSTRUATION CYCLES	59	
DENTAL ANAESTHESIA	59	
DEPRESSION	46	136
DEVIATION OF THE EYE	59	
DEVIATION OF THE MOUTH	59	
DIABETES	59	
DIARRHEA	46	137
DIFFICULTY IN BREATHING	47	138
DIFFICULTY IN SWALLOWING	47	139
DIFFICULTY IN URINATING	47	140
DISCOLORATION OF THE SCLERA	47	141
DIVERTICULITIS	47	142
DIZZINESS	48	143
DROOLING	59	
DROOPING OF THE EYELIDS	59	
DRYNESS OF THE MOUTH	48	145
DRYNESS OF THE TONGUE	48	146
DYSENTERY	48	147
DYSMENORRHEA	49	148
EAR INFECTION	49	150
EARACHE	49	149
EATING DISORDERS	49	151
ECZEMA	49	152
EDEMA	49	153
ELECTRIC AND ELECTROMAGNETIC ENERGY IMBALANCES	50	154
EMOTIONAL CHEST PAIN	43	120
EMPHYSEMA	59	
ENLARGEMENT OF THE BREAST IN MALE	59	
ENVIRONMENTAL TOXICITY/SICK BUILDING SYNDROME	50	155
EPILEPSY	51	160
EPSTEIN-BARR VIRUS	51	161
EXCESSIVE PERSPIRATION	51	162
EXCESSIVE UTERINE BLEEDING	40	104
EYE INFECTIONS	50	157
EYE INFLAMMATION	50	156
EYE PAIN	50	158
EYE STRESS	50	159
FACIAL PALSY	59	
FAILING MEMORY	59	
FAILING VISION	59	
FAINTING	51	163
FALLING EYEBROWS	59	
FALLING HAIR	59	
FAR SIGHTEDNESS	59	
FAT INTOLERANCE	59	
FEAR IN CHILDREN	60	

	Page	Diagram Page
FEAR IN GENERAL	60	
FEAR OF DARKNESS	59	
FEAR OF STRANGERS	59	
FEVER	51	164
FEVER WITHOUT SWEATING	60	
FIBROMYALGIA	52	165
FLATULENCE	60	
FOOD POISONING	52	166
FOOD RETENTION	60	
FORGETFULLNESS	60	
FREQUENCY OF URINATION	60	
FROZEN SHOULDER	60	
GALL BLADDER PAIN	52	168
GASTRIC ULCER	60	
GENERAL BODY ACHE	52	167
GLAUCOMA	60	
HAIR LOSS IN MEN	60	
HAIR LOSS IN WOMEN	60	
HAIR LOSS DUE TO CHEMOTHERAPY	60	
HAND TREMOR	60	
HAY-FEVER	60	
HEADACHES IN GENERAL	53	173
HEART IRREGULARITIES	53	171
HEARTBURN	54	178
HEAT SENSATION IN THE SOLE	52	170
HEAT STROKE	52	169
HEMORRHOIDS, BLEEDING OR IRRITATION	41	106
HICCUP	60	
HIGH BLOOD PRESSURE	54	179
HIGH BLOOD UREA NITROGEN	60	
HIGH CHOLESTEROL IN THE BLOOD	60	
HIGH BLOOD CREATININE	60	
HIGH SODIUM INTAKE	60	
HIGH TRIGLYCERIDES	60	
HIVES	54	180
HOARSE VOICE	60	
HODGKIN'S DISEASE	60	
HORMONE IMBALANCE IN FEMALE	60	
HORMONE IMBALANCE IN MALE	60	
HOT FLASHES	60	
HOT PALMS AND SOLES	60	
HYPERACIDITY	60	
HYPOGLYCEMIA	53	172
IMMATURE BLOOD CELL PRODUCTION	60	
IMMUNE DEFICIENCY DISORDERS	60	
IMPOTENCE	60	
IMPROVE MEMORY	60	
IMPROVE CONCENTRATION	60	
IMPROVE YANG ENERGY IN OLDER PEOPLE	60	
INDIGESTION	55	181
INFERTILITY IN MEN	60	
INSOMNIA	55	182
INTERNAL BLEEDING	60	
IRRITABILITY	60	
ITCHING OF THE WHOLE BODY	60	
ITCHY EYES	60	
JET LAG	60	

Index (contd.)

	Page	Diagram Page
JOCK ITCH	.60	
KIDNEY INFECTION	.60	
KIDNEY NOT ABLE TO FILTER ENOUGH URINE	.60	
LACTATION DEFICIENCY	.61	
LARYNGITIS	.55	183
LEAKY GUT SYNDROME	.55	184
LEUKEMIA	.61	
LIVER FLUKES	.61	
LONG TERM SICKNESS	.61	
LOOSE STOOLS WITH UNDIGESTED FOOD	.61	
LOW ENERGY	.55	185
LOW IMMUNITY	.61	
LOW PLATELETS	.61	
LOW RED BLOOD CELL COUNT	.61	
LOW SEXUAL DESIRE IN MEN	.61	
LOW SEXUAL DESIRE IN WOMEN	.61	
LOW SPERM COUNT	.61	
LOW WHITE BLOOD CELL COUNT	.61	
LOWER ABDOMINAL PAIN	.34	68
LOWER BACKACHE	.38	91
LUMP IN THE THROAT	.61	
LUMPS IN THE BREAST	.61	
LUNG CONGESTION	.43	119
LUPUS ARTHRITIS	.37	88
MACULAR DEGENERATION	.61	
MANIC DISORDERS	.61	
MASTITIS	.61	
MENAPAUSAL DISORDERS	.61	
MENSTRUATION TROUBLE (PMS)	.56	186
MENTAL CLARITY	.61	
MENTAL DISORDERS	.61	
MID BACKACHE	.38	92
MIGRAINES (BLADDER HEADACHES)	.54	177
MIGRAINES (GALL BLADDER HEADACHES)	.53	174
MIGRAINES (LIVER HEADACHES)	.53	175
MIGRAINES (STOMACH HEADACHES)	.54	176
MOOD SWINGS	.61	
MOTOR IMPAIRMENT	.61	
MULTIPLE SCLEROSIS	.61	
MUSCLE SPASMS OF THE UPPER BACK	.61	
MUSCULAR ATROPHY	.61	
MUSCULAR DYSTROPHY	.61	
MUTISM	.61	
MYELITIS	.61	
MYOPIA	.61	
NAUSEA/ Morning sickness	.56	187
NECK PAINS AND STIFFNESS	.61	
NEUROMA	.61	
NEUROTIC VOMITING	.61	
NEVER HAPPY WITH ANYTHING	.61	
NIGHT BLINDNESS	.61	
NIGHT SWEAT	.61	
NIGHTMARES	.48	144
NOCTURNAL EMISSION	.61	
OSTEOARTHRITIS	.61	
OVERACTIVE MIND	.56	188
OVERWEIGHT DUE TO WATER RETENTION	.62	

	Page	Diagram Page
PAIN AND MOTOR IMPAIRMENT OF THE SHOULDER	62	
PAIN AND STIFFNESS OF THE LOWER BACK	62	
PAIN AND SWELLING OF THE DORSUM OF THE FOOT	62	
PAIN AROUND THE UMBILICUS	61	
PAIN BEHIND THE EARS	61	
PAIN IN THE BREAST	61	
PAIN IN THE FACE	61	
PAIN IN THE HEEL	62	
PAIN IN THE HYPOCHONDRIAC REGION	61	
PAIN IN THE LATERAL ASPECT OF THE UPPER ARM	62	
PAIN IN THE SCAPULAR REGION	62	
PAIN IN THE TESTICLE	62	
PAIN IN THE EXTERNAL GENITALIA	61	
PAINFUL INTERCOURSE	62	
PARALYSIS OF THE FOOT	62	
PARALYSIS OF THE LIMBS	62	
POOR DIGESTION OF CARBOHYDRATES	62	
POSTNASAL DRIPS	62	
PREVENT SAGGING BREAST	62	
PREVENT SLEEPING	62	
PROMOTE YAWNING	62	
PRURITUS VULVAE	62	
PSORIASIS	62	
REDUCES FAT FROM THE THIGHS	62	
RESTLESS LEG SYNDROME	56	189
RHEUMATOID ARTHRITIS	37	87
SALIVATION, ABNORMAL	62	
SCIATIC NEURALGIA	56	190
SENSATION OF PLUGGED EAR	62	
SHORTNESS OF BREATH	56	191
SORE THROAT	57	192
SPONTANEOUS SWEATING	62	
SPRAIN ANKLE	62	
STAGE FRIGHT	62	
STERILITY IN WOMEN	62	
SUGAR CRAVING	62	
T.M.J. PAIN	62	
TEARING OF THE EYES	62	
TEMPER TANTRUM IN CHILDREN	62	
TO BOOST UP ENERGY	62	
TO CALM DOWN	62	
TO DECREASE APPETITE	62	
TO INCREASE THE BUST SIZE IN WOMEN	62	
TO LIVE LONG	61	
TO MEND BROKEN HEARTS	62	
TO REDUCE WRINKLES	62	
TOO MUCH SWEATING	62	
TOOTHACHE	57	193
TUNNEL VISION	62	
TWITCHING OF ANY PART OF THE BODY	62	
TWITCHING OF THE EYELIDS	62	
UNABLE TO CRY	57	194
UNHAPPY DISPOSITION	62	
UPPER BACKACHE	62	
VARICOSE VEINS	62	
VERTIGO	62	
WARTS	62	

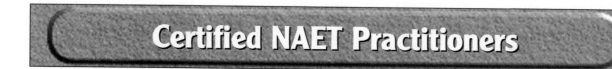
ALABAMA
Gekler, Sandra
Fairhope-(334) 928 8763

ALASKA
Allen, George, D.C
Homer-(907) 235 7221

Trekell, Stanley G. , D.C
Anchorage-(907) 522 1662

Denton, Sandra C., M.D.
Anchorage-(907) 563 6200

Ihlen, Sandy, L.P.N.
Anchorage-(907) 561 6846

Lamothe, Nick, B.S.N.
Anchorage-(907) 562 2672

Marianne Miller, D.C.,
Anchorage-(907) 562 1062

Hoch, Pamela, N.D.
Fairbanks-(907) 456 1858

Krohn, Joyce Ellen L.Ac
Juneau-(907) 586 2577

Lizer, Gerald W. D.C
Eagle River-(907) 694 9535

Barrington, Edward D.C
Anchorage-(907) 562 5366

ARIZONA
Ney, Peter, D.C
Cottonwood-(520) 639 1700

Grade, Thomas, J. M.D
Gilbert-(602) 981 4250

Carlsen, Brete, D.C
Tatcher-(520) 343 9099

Cooper, Carol, L.Ac, L.C.S.W.
Chandler-(602) 777 9045

CALIFORNIA
Chilbert, Christine
Alamo-(510) 838 4361

Yamas, John, L.Ac., OMD
Arcata-(707) 822 7400

Sperry, Shirley S., Ph.D
Auburn-(916) 878 9400

Herrick, Ann L.Ac
Berkeley-(510) 528 9821

Lippman, Cathie-Ann, M.D.
Beverly Hills-(310) 289 8430

Campion, Toby, D.C
Beverly Hills-(310) 273 1221

Nambudripad, Kris., L.Ac.
Buena Park-(714) 523 8900

Moosad, Mala, R.N., L.Ac
Buena Park-(714) 523 8900

Jones, Marilyn, D.C.
Calabasas-(818)-222-2080

Goodkin, Valarie L.Ac., O.M.D.
Carlsbad-(619) 720 2273

Spencer, Gena, L.Ac
Carmichael-(916) 486 9762

Koven, Arianne, N.D
Cathedral City-(619) 328 1070

Barta, Jeanne, D.C.
Concord-(510) 682 4941

Cutler, Ellen, D.C.
Corte Madera-(415) 924 2273

Steve Mackewicz, L.Ac
Corte Madera-(415) 927 1606

Allen Dubner, D.C
Cupertino-(408) 996 1042

David Nelson, Ph.D
Encinitas-(619) 632 9042

Penny Wells, L.Ac
Encinitas-(619) 943 8850

Norton, Mary L.Ac
Fairfax-(415) 485 9242

Dillon, Christine D.C
Fairfax-(415) 454 4650

Kim, Susan, D.C
Fremont-(510) 795 8949

Zeischegg, Peter, D.C.
Grass Valley-(916) 273 1275

Spurgin, Shirley D.C
Hemet-(909) 658 7219

Katz, David L.Ac.
N. Hollywood-(818) 508 6188

Hall, Thomas J., D.C
Irvine-(714) 250 9206

Pallos, Andrew, D.D.S.
Laguna Niguel-(714) 495 6484

Abell, Robert, N.D., L.Ac
Laguna Niguel-(714)831 1340

Ditter, Shelly, R.N., D.C.
So. Lake Tahoe-(916) 542 4476

Tatsuno, Walter, D.C.
La Jolla-(619) 457 0283

Weiner, Neal K., D.V.M.
Lewiston-(916) 778 3109

Chambreau, Marylyn C. D.C
Los Altos-(415) 948 3282

Mike Greenberg, D.C.
Los Angeles-(213) 826 0972

Roya Darvish, L.Ac
Los Angeles-(310) 288 5959

Steele, Jan K, L.Ac., OMD
Los Angeles-(213) 936 3162

Eberstein, Joycelyn, L.Ac.
Los Angeles-(310) 446 1968

Esparza, Moctesuma, B.A. MFA
Los Angeles-(310) 281 3770

Arlo Gordin, D.C
Los Angeles-(213) 438 0303

Bennett, Susanne, D.C
Los Angeles-(310) 446 2199

Smith, Kenneth J., D.C
Mariposa-(209) 966 5634

Feldman, Alice, L.Ac.
Milbrae-(415) 692 1816

Hays, Robin, O.M.D, L.Ac
Milpitas-(408) 946 9332

Cutler, Steve, D.C.
Mill Valley-(415) 383 4700

Bruce Heckard, D.C
Napa-(707) 226 8683

Weir, Irit, L.Ac
Napa-(707) 226 8924

Shu, Steven, L.Ac
Newport Beach-(714) 759 1869

Curry, Mary, L.Ac, O.M.D
Oakland, CA 94619
(510) 530 8886

Doyle, Kathy, D.C
Oakland-(510) 601 6325

Margaret, Joan, D.C
Oakland-(510) 658 9066

Cass, Hyla, M.D.
Pacific Palisades-CA 90272
(310) 459 9866

Lydick, Shannon, L.Ac.
Palm Desert-(619) 776 4599

Hilsdale, Karin, L.Ac.,
Pasadena-(818)-585-8877

Rawlinson, Ian, L.Ac
Petaluma-(707) 762 4309

Herry Hom, L.Ac
Petaluma-(415) 647 6222

Kuss, Timothy, N.D.,
Pleasantville-(800) 733 9293

Lake, Janet, D.C
Pomona-(909) 624 9016

Miliken, Jacqueline, N.D
Rancho Cordova-(916) 635 3772

Smillie, Jaqueline, M.T.
Redlands-(909) 335 1980

Fleming, Tapas E., L.Ac
Redondo Beach-(310) 375 3628

Krestan, Sandy, L.Ac.
Richmond-(510) 237 9952

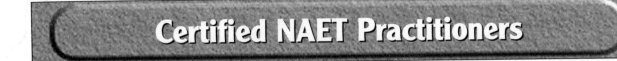
Crystal Sage, N.D
Roseville-(916) 781 3598

J.P.Seckel
Sacramento-(916) 424 0242

Reuben, Carolyn, L.Ac.
Sacramento-(916) 452 5887

Inouye, Stanley, DDS, L.Ac.
Sacramento-(916) 421 2890

Levy, Judith, L.Ac.
Sacramento-(916) 395 5588

Gantt, Roc, L.Ac
Sacramento-(916) 349 9223

Finkbine, Steven, L.Ac.
San Anselmo-(415) 454 6901

DeFino, Michael A., D.C
San Anselmo-(415) 453 1588

Kay Patterson Zabler, M.T.
San Diego-(619) 279 3317

Chin, Eleanor, D.C.
San Francisco-(415) 243 0678

Newmark, Irene, L.Ac
San Francisco-(415) 552 3813

Lewis, Julia, D.C.
San Jose-(408) 526 9423

Cadwallader, Claudia L.Ac
San Luis Obispo-(805) 466 6825

Bunis, Sobyl, D.C
Santa Barbara-(805) 966 3003

Schafer, Paul, D.c
Santa Barbara-(803) 687 1730

Eisen, J. De Rousseau, Ph.D
Santa Barbara-(805) 962 3311

Eisen, Jeffrey, Ph.D,
Santa Barbara-(805) 962 3311

Wolfeld, Joanne, L.Ac
San Mateo-(415) 344 3640

Fitzgerald, Patricia, L.Ac.
Santa Monica -(310) 451-7170

Manzetti, Teresa, D.C.
Santa Monica-(310) 452 9146

Phillips, Gloria, D.C.,
Santa Monica-(310) 458 8020

Nickel, Ruth, L.Ac.
Santa Monica-(310) 392 6751

Fairfield, Peter, L.Ac
San Rafael-(415) 439 4239

Miseveth, Sara, D.C
San Rafael-(415) 453 1040

Thomas, Helen, D.C.
Santa Rosa-(707) 527 7313

Thomas, Craig, D.C.
Santa Rosa-(707) 527 7313

Willens, Randall, L.Ac.
Santa Rosa-(707) 542 1470

Zafis, Cindy, D.C.
Santa Rosa-(707) 579 9550

Walker, Sydney, L.Ac.
Santa Rosa-(707) 544 8802

Gold, Michelle D.C
Santa Rosa-(707) 579 2234

Hope Ryf, L.Ac
Thousand Oaks-(805) 497 4074

Gorrie, David, D.C.
Tustin-(714) 544 9789

Raviv, Hagit, L.Ac.
Van Nuys-(818) 787 8435

Decapua, Jerome, D.C.
Willow Creek-(916)629 2474

Elias, Ann, L.Ac.
Willowcreek-(916) 629 3454

Feldman, Kenneth D.D.S
Woodland Hills-(818) 703 5059

Ernest, Kym H. D.C
Woodland Hills-(818) 704 1662

Meisinger, Susan B., D.C. L.Ac
Woodland Hills-(818) 883 1242

Cesmat, Barbara, D.C.H
Woodland Hills-(818) 703 6212

Bush, Dave, D.C
Woodland Hills-(818) 704 1662

Allen, Corinne, Ph.D
Yorba Linda-(800) 929 2999

CONNECTICUT
Bailey, Richard, D.C., L.Ac
Danbury-(203) 789 9355

Albini, Mary Ellen, L.Ac
Hamden-(203) 585 8164

COLORADO
Corpany, Carol, R.N.
Colorado Spgs-(719) 633 2752

Salsman, William, D.C
Colorado Springs-(719) 579 0180

Culver, Roy, D.C.
Longmont-(303) 651 1234

Messer, Alan R., D.C
Longmont-(303) 776 6110

Cortini, Cynthia, D.C
Englewood-(303) 721 9984

Owens, Beth, L.Ac
Englewood-(303) 770 6704

Hays, David, L., D.C.
Colorado Springs-(719) 570 1208

FLORIDA
Russell, Robert, L.Ac
Miami-(305) 667 8787

Andely, Cynthia, L.Ac
N.Miami Beach-(305) 947 2701

Kufe, Marita, L.Ac
Sarasota-(941) 377 4974

Phillips, Douglas, DDS
West Palm Beach-(561) 848 1720

Drucker, Steven, D.C.
Boca Raton-(561) 392 7989

Holyk, Peter, M.D
Sebastian-(407) 388 1222

Kenemouth, David, D.C
Winterhaven-(941) 294 5399

P.T. Ferrance, A.P
Hollywood-(954) 986 9882

Jones, Lyn, D.C., R.N.
Frostproof-(941) 635 3562

Pollack, Joseph, D.C
W. Palm Beach-(561) 964 6797

Snyder, Gary S., D.C
Ft. Landside-(954) 486 4000

GEORGIA
Koeppel, Heather, D.C
Atlanta-(404) 633 8255

HAWAII
Tavily, Farangis, L.Ac.
PU Hoa-(808) 965 9757

Jones, Molly L.Ac
Kapaa-(808) 822 2884

Connor, Yvonne, M.D.
Wailu Ku-Maui-(808) 249 0124

Christman, Randol, D.Ac.
Maui-(808) 807 9434

Tan, Karen, N.D, L.Ac
Honolulu-(808) 593 9445

Fickes, Linda, D.C
Honolulu-(808) 377 1811

Keller, Sophie, L.Ac
Keaau-(808) 982 9886

Amdur, Latifa, N.D, L.Ac
Hanalei-(808) 828 1155

IDAHO
Cozzi, Robert L.Ac
Sandpoint-(208) 263 4512

Linda Hadley, N.D
Boise-(208) 322 9376

ILLINOIS:
Olson, Pamela, D.C, L.Ac
Elgin-(847) 888 3133

Bain, Alan F., D.O
Chicago-(312) 236 7010

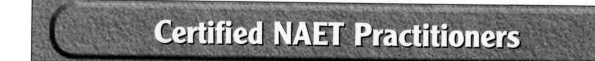

Herazy, Theodore, D.C
Champaign-(217) 352 0808
Baschleben, Jackie, D.C
Roscoe-(815) 623 7694

IOWA
Frogley, Chris J., D.C
DavenPort-(319) 386 4798

Siemsen, Patricia A., R.N
Long Grove-(319) 285 4389

Corn, Suddha Cindi, D.C
Fairfield-(515) 469 9804

INDIANA
Quintero, Suzanne M., DVM
W. Lafayette-(317) 463 9520

KANSAS
Christenson, James L., D.O.
Coffeyville-(316) 251 1100

Martin, Michael, E., D.C
Topeka-(913) 357 5100

KENTUCKY
Konopka, Anthony, L.Ac
Crestwood-(502) 241 8621

MASSACHUSETTS
Sampson, Robert, M.D.
Andover-(978) 474 9009

MARYLAND
Rukus, Monika, L.Ac
Rockville-(301) 881 5980

Norton, Reggi, M.A.C, L.Ac
Gaithersburg-(301) 977 7762

Stearns, Rebecca L., L.Ac
Rockville-(301) 230 1477

Rodriguez, Asher A., D.C
Baltimore-(410) 256 6717

Beals, Paul, M.D
Laurel-(301) 490 9911

Huetter, Janice E., N.D
Hagerstown-(301) 797 7395

Hudson, Helen, M.Ac
Timorium-(410) 252 3197

Camper, Sandy, L.Ac
Columbia-(410) 997 2052

MAINE
Norton, Jody J., D.C
Blue Hill-(207) 374 2186

Tsao, Fern L.Ac
Yarmouth-(207) 846 4433

MICHIGAN
Sauders, Gregory S., Ph.D.
(Acu)
Adrian-(517) 263 3859

Waytula, Ellen, L.Ac.
Lawton-(616) 624 1837

Wechter, Elizbeth, L.Ac
Otsego-(616) 657 8330

Keyte, Steven, D.C
Kalamazoo-(616) 342 0201

Keyte, Gerald, D.O.
Washington-(810) 781 5535

Brownstein, David, M.D
Farmington Hills-(810) 857 1600

MINNESOTA
Caldwell, George S., O.M.D
Mount-(612) 422 9910

Muedeking, Nancy, P.T
Bloomington-(612) 881 3045

NEVADA
Hetzel, David D.C
Henderson-(702) 260 1164

Carol Alexander
Las Vegas-(702) 227 5725

NEW JERSEY
Huber, Scott P., D.C.
Maplewood-(201) 761 1153

Hokenson, Nancy, R.N., L.Ac
Titusville-(609) 730 0700

San Paolo, Carman Ann, R.N.
Trenton-(609) 581 9005

Nozek, Glenn, D.C
Tom River-(908) 255 0600

Clinton, Nohoma, Ph.D
Princeton-(609) 924 8455

NEW MEXICO
Diaz, Maria, L.Ac, O.M.D.,
Santa Fe-(505) 984 0928

Krohn, Jacqueline A., M.D
Los Alamos-(505) 662 9620

Bartnett, Beatrice D.C, N.D
Ruidoso-(505) 258 3046

Easton, Jade
Santa Fe-(505) 983 9133

Taylor, Frances A, M.A
Los Alamos-(505) 662 9620

Chernoff, Marilyn,
M.A,N.D,I.D
Albuquerque-(505) 292 2222

NEW YORK
Abrams, Judyth, L.Ac
Ithaca-(607) 277 7713

Cutler, Deborah, D.C.
New York-(212) 741 6285

H.S. Khalsa, L.AC
New York, NY 10003

Roth, Eric, M.D.
New York-(212) 253 0017

Hackman, Robert, L.Ac
Ithaca-(607) 272 5450

NORTH CAROLINA
Kasler, John, D.C.
Charlotte-(704) 537 3823
Prince, Robert, M.D.
Charlotte-(704) 537 0221

OHIO
Christenson, Elizabeth C., M.D
Maumee-(419) 893 8438

OREGON:
Kibert, Ron, D.C.
Portland-(503) 245 3444

Dyler, Shaun, N.D., L.Ac
Tigard-(503) 579 6385

Johnson, Shelly S., L.Ac.
Brookings-707 465 4114

Edie Page, L.Ac
Portland-(503) 222 2235

Gregory K. Doss, O.M.D
Grants Pass-(503) 476 4611

Lori Paiken, L.Ac
Ashland-(503) 488 3612

Marilyn Brewer, L.Ac
Portland-(503) 246 0103

Macelle Chiasson, M.D
Portland-(503) 245 3156

Marc Gadoua, M.L.Ac
Portland-(503) 295 3647

Laura Liggett, L.Ac
Portland-(503) 233 9079

Mathew Sheehan, D.C
Medford-(541) 773 1321

Robert Wilson, N.D
Hood River-(541) 386 5505

Shiela Moran, N.D. L.Ac
Portland-(503) 222 7174

Suzette Taylor, M.T
Portland-(503) 293 1488

Jean Dugan, L.Ac
Milwaukie-(503) 241 5382

Dick Thom, D.D.S, N.D
Beaverton-(503) 520 8859

Dawn Nowlin, L.Ac
Portland-(503) 227 3828

Jeanette Dodge, L.Ac
Portland-(503) 297 7656

Rayna Jacobson, L.Ac, R.N.
Portland-(503) 236 9609

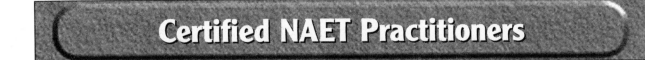

Patrice Peterson, L.Ac
Eugene-(541) 343 5004

Gilda Taylor, R.N.
Portland-(503) 238 8097

Ellen Shefi, L.Ac
Portland-(503) 297 7656

Thomas C. Richards, Ph.D, D.C
Beaverton-(503) 526 8600

Steven Arvidson, N.D
Newberg-(503) 920 3965

Debra L. Martin, N.D
Eugene-(541) 683 4071

Julia Fuller, L.Ac
Portland-(503) 626 6379

Engleman, Carol Sue, N.D
Lake Oswego-(503) 624 7362

Rothstein Lilijoy, D.C
Portland-(503) 294 1235

PENNSYLVANIA
Kerry, Roy E., M.D.
Greenville-(412)-588-9709

Cathy Lynn Goldstein, L.Ac
Fountainville-(215) 230 4600

Sandi Radomski,
Philadelphia-(215) 745 7131

Sandy Steinman, M.Ac
Lancaster-(717) 581 0351

Don M. Weiss, D.C
Philadelphia-(215) 728 1414

Linda Silva, L.Ac
Wyndmoor-(215) 233 1733

Robert Radomski, D.C
Philadelpiha-(215) 745 7131

Richard M. Cassidy, C.A
Washington Crossing-(215) 493 9077

Cara Frank, R.Ac
Philadelphia, PA 19144
(215) 438 2977

Scheckenbach, Mary Ellen L.Ac
Phila-215 438 2595

Thomas, Cherie L. D.C
Avis-(717) 753 8311

Hannah, Suvarna, N.D
Elkins Pk-(215) 579 0409

Gayle Materna, R.N. B.S.N, M.P.H
Lancaster-(717) 560 9300

David Molony, L.Ac
Catasauqua-(610) 264 2755

Roeshman, Robert M., D.O
Allentown-(610) 820 9668

TENNESSEE
Jill Loraine Mc Gregor, L.Ac
Chattanooga-(423) 892 9567

TEXAS
Gary Trott, OMD
Bedford-(817) 285 0622

Danny D. Dore, M.T
Houston-(713) 528 3658

Wiseman, Champion, D.C.
Austin-(512) 465 5374

J.D. Chandler, N.D
Dallas-(214) 340 3342

Jones, Kimberly, D.C
Dallas-(972) 789 1234

Peck, Iva Liu, R.N. L.Ac
Dallas-(214) 380 9070

UTAH
Anderson, Thomas, D.C
Holladay-(801) 272 9989

Mallon, Mary, R.N
Sandy-(801) 495 2603

Clausen, Natalie, L.Ac
Salt Lake City-(801) 359 2705

Sherman, Tom, D.C
Salt Lake City-(801) 967 6000

WASHINGTON
Randy Sandaine, N.D
Colville-(509) 684 1104

Crystal Tack, N.D, C.A
Sequim-(360) 683 2937

D'Vorah R. Levy, M.Ac, L.Ac
Seattle-(206) 324 8600

Augusto Romano, L.Ac
Kent-(206) 852 2866

Merrilee Nelson, R.N.
Puyallup-(206) 840 2794

Ann Mc Combs, D.O
Bellevue-(206) 451 3159

Walter J. Crinnion, N.D
Bellevue-(206) 747 9200

Heather Roberts, N.D
VanCouver-(360) 694 1015

Michelle Gienger, R.N.
Renton-(206) 271 4850

Griffith, Mary, N.D
Gig Harbor-(206) 851 7550

Scott, Anne D., N.D
Vancouver-(300) 750 4642

Hatfield, Lon, M.D
Colville-(509) 684 3701

Terry, Kevin L., D.C
Puyallup-(206) 845 0543

Christiansen, Mary, D.C
Puyallup-(206) 535 6069

Petronelli, Beatrice N.D
Puyallyp-(206) 845 6202

Kitaeff, Richard, N.D.,L.Ac
Edmonds-(206) 775 6001

Areste, Que N.D
Seattle-(206) 328 2926

Phillips, Cindy N.D
Seattle-(206) 726 0034

Whittaker, Melanie N.D
Everett-(206) 290 5309

Bentz, James, D.C
Bellevue-(206) 746 4045

Spencer, Gregory W.,D.P.M.
Renton-(206) 255 7731

Schuck, Herbert I., N.D
Tukwila-(206) 248 0061

Hawkins, Heidi M., L.Ac
Seattle-(206) 285 7363

Lingren, Ardith, M.A.
Woodinville-(206) 483 9699

Mc Donald, Beth, N.D
Everett-(206) 252 7263

Huntley, Susan, R.N
Metaline Fall-(509) 684 3701

Ruppert, Patricia, R.N.
Puyallup-(206) 770 1988
Tangeman, Roger, DC
Spokane-(509) 468 2102

Kennedy, Thomas, M.D
Puyallup-(206) 770 5504

WISCONSIN
Sadof, Miriam, L.Ac
Wanwatosa-(414) 258 5522

Kadile, Eleazar M., M.D.
Green Bay-(414) 468 9442

Weber, Maureen, L.Ac
Fontana-(414) 549 7946

Clements, Melody D.C.
Williams Bay-(414)245 6051

Ensweiler, Mark S., L.Ac, D.C
Plover-(715) 345 0655

Cubbs, Mary Lee, D.C
Milwaukee-(414) 967 9000

Smolen, Frances, M.,
Wanpaca-(715) 258 2313

AUSTRIA/EUROPE
Magrutsch, Edda, N.D.
A-3400 Weidling
Tel. 02243/26576
Tel. 02243/26576
Fax. 02243/ 31991

Hannelore Schrogendorefer, Ac,
A4020 Linz
Austria, Europe

ISRAEL
Shaul, Ofira, L.Ac.
K. ONO 55203
ISRAEL
Tel.03-535 5721

Samuel Hendler, M.D.
Tel Aviv 64381, Israel
Tel.03-5226166

Helena Segal, M.D
Rishon Lezion,
Israel 75215
Tel.9 72 3 9644929